THE
ORANGE
BOOK

A Method of
Self-Realisation

The Study Society

ISBN 978-0-9561442-6-3

First Published 1981 by
The Society for the Study of Normal Psychology,
Colet House, 151 Talgarth Road, London W14 9DA
Telephone: 020 8748 9338, Fax: 020 8563 0551
email: office@studysociety.org
Website: www.studysociety.org

Reprinted 2002, 2006, 2012
Translation: Spanish: Mexican Study Group 2000

Printed in England by:
The Vale Press
Willersey, Worcestershire,
WR12 7RR

FOREWORD

This volume is a kind of textbook of how to put into practice the realisation of Unity (Self-Realisation); it is complete in itself and requires no other methods. In fact it will appear to be contrary to the point of view and the methods recommended in any other available source; and yet it demonstrates the real meaning of many enigmatic sayings by great teachers. A single reading is insufficient; to obtain the real benefit one must live with the contents of this book, continually trying to find a way to practise what it says.

A full definition and description of the idea of 'Param-Atman' is to be found on the first few pages of the main text. However, it should be explained briefly that the word Atman signifies the individual Self, while the term Param-Atman means Universal Self, of which the Atman is an 'atom' of the same substance with all the same properties. This idea lifts the student above all confusion which arises over the perennial question: What can I call 'I', in the sense of a permanent entity within my ever-changing nature?

F. C. Roles

Collected together in this volume is a distillation of knowledge the implications of which have scarcely yet been explored. I find myself drawn to return to these words again and again, and never fail to find new refreshment. They can be recommended to anyone who feels there are questions unanswered.

M. J. Harris
Chairman, Wellington Study Group Inc.
New Zealand

The Shankaracharya

His Holiness Shantanand Saraswati was Shankaracharya of Jyotir Math in Northern India from 1953 until his retirement in 1980. His Holiness, who came from the ancient Advaita or nondualist tradition of knowledge and meditation, was one of India's greatest saints. He continued the work of his predecessor, His Holiness Brahmananda Saraswati (Gurudeva), in making mantra meditation available to people of many religious traditions.

Translators

'D' and 'RLD' appear quite often. They refer to Shri R. L. Dixit who lived in Allahabad and was a devotee of HH. He often attended our audiences and occasionally acted as interpreter. He very kindly made notes and sent us transcripts of talks HH gave at his Ashram, and at the great annual religious festival – the Mela. This book is composed mainly of the talks sent by Shri Dixit. Other material was translated by Shri S. M. Jaiswal and Shri Narayan Swaroop Agrawal.

Appendix

An appendix of additional material from the Shankaracharya, expanding on the ideas of Bhakti, the Gunas, Cosmic Laws and the concept of surrender and sacrifice has been added to this edition.

CONTENTS

During the Autumn of 1970, the Shankaracharya spoke several times to the people at his Ashram in Allahabad on the subject of *Param-Atman* (Universal Self).

This was the first translation we received.

DISCOURSE ON MEDITATION AND PARAM-ATMAN
By His Holiness the Shankaracharya

August 1970

Meditation, meditator, and the object of meditation, these three always go together. There can be no meditation if either the meditator or the object of meditation are not there. The object of meditation is *Param-Atman*, the Ultimate Truth, the Absolute Truth, and the One and Only Truth that has Real Existence.

There is no such thing as the 'World'† from the point of view of real existence. Yet we see a 'world' around us. This seeing is like seeing a mirage, seeing a thing where there is none.

Unreal though a mirage is, we cannot dispel it by any physical means. That is, we cannot dig it out with a spade or blow it away with artillery. As it is due to certain conditions of light, it goes away only when those conditions have gone. Similarly, the mirage of the 'world' is due to certain conditions of ignorance, and it goes away only when that ignorance is gone.

---

†Used in the same sense as Christ's words, 'In the world ye will have tribulation, but be of good cheer, I have overcome the world.'

Consider a sugar cube; the real thing about it is its sweetness. Its form is irrelevant – whether it is cubical or round or any other shape. Now the *Manas* ('computer mind') is incapable of imagining 'sweetness', though it is real. It can, however, imagine objects having the property of sweetness – like a sugar cube or fruit or pudding; and these, in turn, enable us to realise what sweetness is. Thus to get at the abstract we take the help of the concrete; to get at the extra-sensory we go from the sensory object. Similarly, we meditate with the help of a 'mantra', which is a sensation of sound, in order to get at something which is otherwise beyond the reach of the human mind – the *Param-Atman*.

Let us revert to the sugar cube. The sugar cube comes from sugar; sugar comes from sugar cane; sugar cane comes from soil, water, air, light, etc. Carrying on the argument 'this comes from that, that comes from that. . .', we ultimately trace the origin of the sugar cube to the '*Avyakta*' ('Unmanifest Nature'). Then the origin of the sugar cube, which we can perceive through our senses, lies in *Avyakta* which we never could perceive through our senses. Similarly, all perceptible phenomena (collectively called 'the world') originated from *Avyakta*, and will finally merge into *Avyakta*. This is the view of the Tradition of the Shankaracharyas.

We want to think about the *Param-Atman*. As it is the source of all greatness, its own greatness must be infinite. As it is the source of all happiness, its own happiness must be boundless. As it is the source of all beauty, its own beauty must be – we do not know. . . But how could we ever think about such a *Param-Atman* whose qualities and nature are thus beyond the utmost stretch of human imagination?

This was the question which was naturally put by Arjuna to the Lord Krishna, and the answer is contained in the *Bhagavad Gita*, chapter 10, verses 20–42.

Here is a translation of a few of those verses:

> O Arjuna, I am the Self, seated in the hearts of all beings, I am the beginning, and the life, and I am the end of them all.

> Of the scriptures I am the hymns; I am the electric force in the powers of nature; of the senses, I am the registering mind; and I am the intelligence in all that lives.

> Among the vital forces I am life itself; I am Mammon to the heathen and godless; I am energy in fire, earth, wind, heaven, sun, moon and planets. . .

> I am all-devouring Death; I am the origin of all that may happen; I am fame, fortune, speech, memory, intellect, constancy and forgiveness.

> I am the gambling of the cheat, and the splendour of the splendid; I am victory; I am effort; I am the purity of the pure. . .

> Whatever is glorious, excellent, beautiful or mighty, be assured that it comes from only a part of My splendour.

> But what is the use of all these details to you? O Arjuna! I sustain all this world with only a fragment of Myself.

All this implies that by thinking of the most powerful manifest thing as only a tiny particle of *Param-Atman*'s power; by thinking of the most beautiful object we can, and then treating it as a mere atom of the *Param-Atman's* beauty, and so on, we can gradually find our way to the *Param-Atman*. Thus, starting from sensory objects and rising higher and higher, we reach a state where all difference between sensory and ultra-sensory, between definable and indefinable has faded away from us.

Then, what to ordinary people are *different* forms and shapes, are to a Fully-Realised person all manifestations of one and the same *Param-Atman*. What he sees then, around himself and within himself, is *Param-Atman*, and *not* the mirage which we call 'the world'. Such a man would welcome heat and cold, pleasure and pain, fortune and misfortune – all alike, because all are manifestations of *Param-Atman*.

30 August 1970
Reply from His Holiness to questions from FCR

Is there any further advice His Holiness can give on the subject that the Atman alone is real and looks on all the changing events and situations as a passing show, without getting involved?

HH: In order to appreciate the Self described in the *Upanishads*, one needs simple methods. Many such descriptions have been given in the past, but more light can now be thrown on the subject. The states of consciousness experienced in deep sleep, dreams, the day-time state, spiritual awakening, *Samadhi*, etc., are governed by the influx of *Sattva, Rajas* and *Tamas* from people, situations and events. These all undergo change, but the Observer

4

who sees them all as a 'passing show' remains always the same. This Observer never registers any change in itself, if any modification appears, then this must happen to the individual ego ('*Ahankara*') since change is its very nature...

For example, pure gold always remains gold while its uses and shapes and forms are liable to many modifications. The sky remains the same while storms, clouds, rain and snow keep on changing our view of it, and yet do not affect the sky in any way. *(One experiences this vividly every time a plane takes us up above the cloud ceiling.)* The waves of the sea cause no loss or gain to it. In the same way all these passing shows of the *Gunas* do not change the *Atman*, but only provide variety in its appearance.

20 October 1970
Letter from D to FCR

I had a brief talk with His Holiness about how you have tried to explain *Param-Atman* to your group – 'The sum total of all the Atmans of all individual living beings, past, present and to come is *Param-Atman*.'

His Holiness said:
In a way, you can think like that. But you might add that:

1. *Param-Atman* is the *Atman* of the whole universe –
   living and non-living, conceivable and inconceivable.

2. *Atman* is the image of the *Param-Atman*, possessing all the
   properties of the *Param-Atman*, just as a mental image of the
   sun can encompass all the properties of the sun such as
   heat, light, etc.

3. The *Atman*, in association with the *Buddhi* (impure), may seem to be under worldly bondage (such as the mind-body machine), but *Param-Atman* is beyond all such things.

19 November 1970
Answer to a letter from DC dated 7 November

Question:
In the children's game of seeking the treasure, or hunt the thimble, with the child blindfolded, we say 'hot' or 'cold' to guide them to the treasure. In my search for the *Atman* I would like someone to say 'hot' or 'cold' to guide my steps. My passion is increasing to recognise the *Atman*.

HH: In the *Antahkarana* of each person, there lives the *Param-Atman* along with the *Jiva-Atman* for the purpose of guidance. Therefore, we get a guiding voice from time to time when we are in difficulties. In order to hear that inner voice we should pray to the all-knowing *Param-Atman* in solitude with a settled mind. Then an answer, to bring us face to face with success, is sure to come forth. To those maintaining a special relationship with the *Param-Atman*, the *Param-Atman* sometimes reveals Himself in a special form in the external world. Therefore, what we have to do is to take guidance in our *Antahkarana* from that immense source of power, the *Param-Atman*, with fullest concentration of mind and humility. If we do so, then the question of hunting for treasure with eyes blindfolded would not arise.

You (DC) have said, 'But my efforts seem ineffectual. Like digging a very large field... It sometimes seems a spade is not enough – a tractor is required!'

On this point His Holiness observes as follows:

After all, the field you speak of is by no means too large for the *Buddhi*. All fields are smaller than *Buddhi*, all lying within the area of *Manas*; yet both of them, together with the power of the *Atman appear* small, and *we* feel small in every field of life. If, instead, we feel that we are great, we are infinite, and all possible fields come within our own *Manas* and *Buddhi*, then our *Manas* and *Buddhi* give an appropriate decision on each problem at once. But this is possible only if we do not try to restrict or to imprison the *Manas* and the *Buddhi* in this small body.

Atman contains *Buddhi*, *Buddhi* contains *Manas* and *Manas* contains the body. But ordinary people think the other way round, i.e. that it is the *body* which contains all that. Here lies the mistake. The moment we take a broad view of our *Manas* and *Buddhi*, the whole universe goes into it.

The manager of an estate gets on well only by listening to the voice of the proprietor. Similarly, for a body-bearing individual, it is beneficial to recognise the voice of the *Param-Atman* that lives in his *Antahkarana*. People endowed with higher intelligence recognise the voice of the *Param-Atman*. Ordinary people can get this guidance through prayers and solitude. And this guidance can solve the hardest of problems. The small spade you mention is, after all, a child of the 'big iron'. If it calls for the help of the 'big iron' that help would not be denied in view of the relationship between the two. Then the small spade would do the work of the tractor all right!

A story illustrates how great powers come to help the small in the event of a firm determination:

A pair of birds lived by the seashore and laid their eggs on a high rock. One day huge waves arose and washed the eggs away. The birds were very much pained at this uncalled-for act of cruelty on the part of the sea, and they made up their minds to fill it up. They took a little seawater in their beaks and dropped it on land, and took a little sand from the land and dropped it into the sea. They did this from morning till evening and day after day.

One day a great saint named Agastya appeared there and he asked them how they hoped to fill up the sea with such attempts.

The birds replied that, since the sea had swept away their children without any provocation, they would go on trying to fill up the sea all their lives. Even after death they would wish to be born again and again to continue that work until it was completed.

The saint was surprised and impressed with such a firm determination on the part of those two tiny birds. As he had supernatural powers to dry up the sea, he ordered it to return the birds' eggs at once. The waves deposited the eggs back on the rock.

This is just a fairy story. Now we shall examine what represents what here. The saint was *Param-Atman*. The birds were man. The sea was the world. And man's true and firm aspirations were the eggs. When man (the birds of the story) sets himself on a true and unshakable purpose, then the *Param-Atman* (the saint) gives him full assistance, and problems (the waves of the sea) bow down in submission.

January 1971
Observation and question from FCR

On this last visit, by about our seventh talk I had begun to be really tired of myself and with my lack of practice, so I said: 'At a very early talk with you eight years ago, you said, 'After constant meditation and work on oneself, the adept starts to realise that a man is not just flesh and bones, but he is also *Antahkarana*, he is Consciousness, and he is Bliss. When he has fully Realised this, everything becomes very simple for him. Whatever he does, the *way* he moves, the *way* he talks, is quite fitting to the dignity of *Atman* (Divine Self). But this stage comes only after full Realisation!'

I went on to say: 'Though this has stayed with me ever since, why has this simple aim taken more than eight years to achieve in spite of all the wonderful help received? Is one just too stupid to succeed?'

His Holiness said cheerfully:
Those eight years have not been wasted, for a good thing has now become known. In this work on Spirit, there can never be a time limit for full Realisation. It depends on the state (at the outset) of the *Antahkarana* (inner nature) of the individual. If that is ready-made at a high level, then Realisation is very quick, otherwise the Realisation will not come about until the cleansing process is complete. It may well take ten or twenty years for some people.

What takes the time is that the knowledge of such ideas must first be appreciated enough to put it into practice – such as the idea which was taken by your *Buddhi* (i.e. intellectually only) that the flesh, bones, *Manas, Antahkarana, are not the Self.* For these relate to the five sheaths described by the first Shri Shankara in *The Crest Jewel*, and anyone will have to penetrate through these sheaths and detach one after another by faithful practice, in order to realise the Self.

Unless this theoretical knowledge, which at most is just good information, is put into constant and continuous use, it never becomes real or Realised Knowledge. And only when that Knowledge is Realised does the individual become Realised.

7 March 1971
Ashram Talk

His Holiness said:
Teaching a thing without knowing it fully does more harm than good. In Allahabad there is a mushroom growth of Sanskrit schools, but there are not enough good teachers to staff them. As such, they only depopularize Sanskrit instead of popularizing it. Thus people stop going to them, resulting in more teachers than pupils. Such schools harm the very cause for which they exist.

A whole lot of rubbish is contained in our very behaviour. One whose behaviour is like that, how could his destiny be otherwise? We should improve our own behaviour first. We should meditate on the *Param-Atman*. This would make us clean internally and externally. People would think of you as they see you. If they see you clean, they would think that you are clean, and they might try to learn cleanliness from you. The qualities of a Self Realised man are given in Chapter 14, verses 19–27 of the *Bhagavad Gita*. But before reaching that stage, practice is required. A new recruit in the army cannot march in step with the others, but after practice he can march in step with a large contingent of soldiers without any difficulty at all. We need not worry too much if we go wrong, but what is important is that we should not form a habit of going wrong. Once we decide not to go wrong again, we are well on the right path. Once we apply ourselves to the *Param-Atman* with a single-minded devotion, we reach the stage of a *Mahatma* in no time and attain permanent peace – as stated in Chapter 9, verses 29–31 of the *Bhagavad-Gita*:

29 I am the same to all beings; to me there is none either hateful or dear. But those who worship Me are in Me and I, too, am in them.[†]

30 Even a bad man, if he begins to worship Me with single-pointed devotion, is seen to be good; for he has formed a holy resolution.

31 Soon does he attain virtue and eternal peace. O Arjuna, know for certain that no devotee of Mine is ever destroyed.

If once during our lifetime an unshakable faith in *Param-Atman* is established, that is, that we belong to the *Param-Atman* and *Param-Atman* belongs to us – then we are out of reach of all harm. At that stage things change their properties for us, a harmful drug becoming harmless. This is how a cup of deadly poison given to

---

[†]Compare St John, Chapter 15:

'Now ye are clean through the word which I have spoken unto you. Abide in Me and I in you ... If ye abide in Me, and My words abide in you, ye shall ask what ye will, and it shall be done unto you.'

Mira, a perfect devotee, lost all its poisonous properties in her hands. We know that substances change their properties during a chemical reaction, i.e. on a chemical plane. Then, why can this not happen on a more subtle plane where much more powerful forces come into play? *Bhakti* (devotion) can do all that. It cleanses you, purifies you, decorates you, and presents you before the *Param-Atman* at your best.

May 1972
Translation of a talk sent to DBC

Gokarna says in the *Shrimad Bhagavatam*: 'This body is only flesh and bones; cease to be attached to it.'

Transfer your attachment to the *Atman*. Because *Atman* is part of the *Param-Atman*, there is no difference between the two. Both are able to cut worldly bondage.

This body is the vehicle and the *Atman* is the rider. Treat the rider separately from the vehicle. It is not easy to do so. It requires years of practice. We practise by thinking this body is God's property, not ours. This mind is God's property, not ours; everything is God's, and nothing is ours. In this way we free ourselves from all attachments, all constraints. Again, this concept is difficult for those who think that 'I' is the physical body.

A Mahatma wished to live in complete solitude, in order that he could meditate undisturbed at all times. He recounted his wish to a rich man. The rich man had an isolated rest-house deep in the forest, rarely visited by mankind. He offered the rest-house to the Mahatma, and in addition provided a young servant to look after his comforts.

The young servant looked after his master so well that his heart was moved. He asked the young servant if he was content with his life, and if he could do anything to bring him happiness. The young man replied that he himself was content and happy, but he was afraid that his dead father had not achieved Self Realisation as he was frequently appearing in his dreams. He asked the Mahatma for a remedy.

During the ensuing nights, the Mahatma was haunted by the problem of the young man's father. One evening, the boy went to a neighbouring village to attend a marriage feast, telling the Mahatma that he would not return until the following morning. So the Mahatma locked up the house and went to bed. Now, the young servant's bed was beside that of the Mahatma and lay empty. The Mahatma's mind was filled with thoughts about the young man's father, and the failure to achieve Self Realisation. He was quite unable to sleep in peace.

The marriage feast was over by midnight, so the boy returned to the house immediately instead of waiting until the morning. When he got back, he climbed over the wall and through the window and fell asleep on his own bed.

At 3.30 in the morning, the Mahatma awoke and saw the bed was occupied. In the darkness he thought that the occupant must be the boy's father (who had been haunting his son's dreams because he had not achieved Self-realisation). He recited holy mantras and sprinkled blessed water over the body, but the boy did not wake up as he was in so deep a sleep. Now the Mahatma became frightened out of his wits, opened the window and jumped out in order to get away. In his haste he fell over with a heavy thud. The noise awakened the young servant. He chased after the Mahatma with a heavy staff thinking that he was a burglar escaping. Eventually they recognised each other before many blows were sustained, and the misunderstanding was cleared up.

In such a way, just a momentary thought stealing unconsciously into the mind, will make its home there; then it appears later at some inopportune moment to cause much mischief. Reels and reels of such thoughts from thousands of years (in many lifetimes) are lying printed in our minds. They will not let us have peace, unless we develop the same attachment towards God as we have towards the world.

Our desires (wishes) are like so many strings that pull us towards the world.† Let this pull be towards God, instead of towards the world. The method is to think (see) that everything, including one's physical body and mind, belongs to God. Whatever actions we do, including eating, drinking, reading, writing and looking after our duties, should all be dedicated to God.

Bhagavad Gita, chapter 9, verse 26:

> He who offers to Me with devotion only a leaf or a
> flower, or a fruit, or even a little water, this I accept from
> that yearning soul, because with a pure heart it was
> offered with love.

This is the meaning of *Bhakti* (yoga of Devotion). Done in this way, each and every action of yours becomes an act of devotion and so becomes an act of worship to God, instead of being a worldly engagement. The worldly ties then are broken, and the presence of God supervenes.

---

†P D Ouspensky: 'Man is a marionette pulled by invisible strings.'

In the absence of such a mode of thought, there is the world, and with the world there is all our trouble!

7 May 1971
Address by His Holiness at Allahabad

Vyasa says, 'I have made a critical study of the *Vedas* and the *Shastras* several times. The gist of all that, as I have found, is that we should think of the *Param-Atman* at all times.'

As soon as any other thought enters the mind, we are in the grip of *Maya* or 'ignorance', which catches hold of us and takes us very, very far away.

The *Jiva*, or our 'Self', is a part of the *Param-Atman*, and it has come into the world for the sake of discovering joy. But, instead of that, *it has fallen into the trap of ignorance. Ignorance is forgetting the Reality.* It is the root cause of all the troubles associated with the world. Therefore the biggest of all the troubles is to forget the Reality. And, by forgetting the Reality, we mean forgetting that only *Param-Atman* is real and the world is unreal.

A schoolboy was given a new penknife by his parents for his birthday, and he took it to school with him. Usually he carried his penknife in his satchel, but that day he wore the new one in his belt. But when he wanted it, he forgot that it was in his belt, and searched for it again and again in his satchel. Not finding it, he thought his classmates had stolen it, and reported the theft to the class teacher. The whole class was punished. This is how a most ordinary instance of forgetting causes big trouble.

All worldly objects are like children's toys – a toy elephant, a toy motor car, a toy locomotive, etc. They must be treated as nothing more than toys. Disappointments and trouble will be our lot if we treat them as real.

A village landlord was counting some rupee coins which he had earned that day. His little children happened to come and ask for the coins to play with. He asked them to wait till the next day, when he promised to give them better and brighter rupees. The children agreed, and he went to a potter and asked him to prepare 500 earthen rupee coins, painting them bright. The potter promised to deliver them the next day.

The next day the landlord went again to the potter and asked, 'Now, would you give me my 500 rupees?'

The potter replied, 'Not today, if you don't mind; please collect them tomorrow.'

Other customers standing there had heard this conversation between the potter and the landlord. The landlord called them to his house and said, 'You have heard our conversation. I asked the potter to let me have my 500 rupees, and he said that he would do so the next day. I am going to file a suit for the recovery of this amount and you stand witness.'

The suit was filed and the potter lost the case. Thus unreal rupees caused some real trouble.

Similarly, unreal worldly objects cause real troubles, and these end as soon as we know the Reality.

During a juggler's show a juggler strewed the ground with currency notes, while he himself was on contract at

Rs 50/- per day only. People were amused to see such a profusion of currency notes, but none took them seriously as they knew that they were of no value. All worldly objects around us are like that.

The first of the *Upanishads* (*Isha Upanishad*) begins:

'Whatever lives is full of the Lord. Claim nothing; enjoy, do not covet His property. Then hope for a hundred years of life doing your duty.'

They do not ask us to live a hundred years of misery. However, our life does become a life of misery because of our feeling of *attachment* to worldly objects, and this feeling of attachment to worthless things is the root of all miseries. The world, as such, has no miseries at all. It is we who manufacture them by harbouring an attachment to worldly objects.

Attachment means, to consider as 'ours' what really belongs to God. Our body, our house, our wealth, our son, etc. Give up this feeling, and you get rid of all troubles.

Do not think that the world around you, i.e., your house, your money, your body, etc, are unsubstantial. Rather, it is your feeling of attachment to them that is unsubstantial. Whatever is happening around you is right, but what is wrong about it is the *view* you are taking of it. If you could correct your viewpoint, you would be happy.

The world is a great show, which God is staging around you in the shape of the universe. But it is a mere show. Your birth is a show, your death is a show. Actually there is neither birth nor death. Know that, and you would be happy.

The common outlook is that the world is everything, and that *Param-Atman* is nothing. It is a crime to hold this view, and the punishment for it is to be imprisoned in this physical body. You cannot be happy while undergoing a term of imprisonment.

Our mind has the property of thinking of something or other all the time; it cannot remain idle. If it does not remember the *Param-Atman*, it would think of the world. Remembering the *Param-Atman* leads to happiness, and thinking of the world leads to unhappiness.

It is true that people do not find it easy to hold the *Param-Atman* in mind. The reason for that is lack of practice. As long as the ability has not been acquired, there would be difficulty. But the ability can certainly be acquired.

A baby cannot eat solid food at the beginning because the ability has not been acquired. But this ability comes quite easily later when he tries (after he has some teeth!).

Acquiring the ability to think of the *Param-Atman* is as easy as that.

> Someone went to a Mahatma and said that he would like to serve him, but he added that he must have something to do all the time as he could not remain idle. The Mahatma asked him to go and cut a long piece of bamboo. When he did so, he asked him to fix it in the ground. This done, he asked him to climb to the top of it, then come down, climb again, come down again, and so on. Thus he had constant work to do.

Similarly, keep the mind occupied, otherwise you would go mad.

You have a mind, you have a body, and you have intelligence. Let the mind be trained to remember the *Param-Atman*, let the body do service to Him, and let the intelligence discriminate.

Hari – OM – Tat – Sat

11 June 1971
Evening talk by His Holiness in Allahabad

There is something or other in all of us, which is special or outstanding. For example, some are intelligent, some are unintelligent, some are strong and some are weak, some are learned and some are ignorant, some are rich and some are poor.

Each should try to please God (or serve God, or worship God, as the case may be) with that attribute in which one chiefly excels. This is the path of least resistance. It is sure to work, it has always done so in the past.

> Sudama was the poorest of the poor. He worshipped Krishna with rotten rice only and that, too, was borrowed, because he was so poor. But this worship worked and Sudama got great wealth in return.

Little things are no longer little when consequences become great. In fact, all great things begin from a little.

> A tiny seed of Babul (a thorny tree in India) will produce a large thorny tree at first, then this will immediately produce others until the whole place becomes full of them and nobody can move through without getting hurt.

Similarly, a little wrong action can cause much harm, and a little good action just the opposite.

> Kubja, a hump-backed woman who lived in the time of Krishna, worshipped Krishna with sandalwood paste only, but with total sincerity. All her troubles disappeared, and the hump also went. She became a beautiful woman. Her action was small, but her sincerity was great. Therefore this miracle happened.

Similarly many stories in the *Puranas* illustrate the fact that even the lowest can reach the greatest heights.

The method is: do what each of you is meant for, and do it in a spirit of service to God. Let eating, drinking, sleeping, bathing, etc, all be dedicated to God. This is the correct worship, and the correct *Bhakti*.

> Shabari, an uneducated woman of the *Ramayana* time, worshipped in this way for 100 years in full faith that the personified God would visit her in the jungle one day, and it actually happened. Rama did go to her hut during His exile.

Though illiterate, her dedication was of a higher order than that of even Mahatmas. Therefore, He visited her hut, and not theirs.

> In the epic *Mahabharata*, we read that Krishna declined the invitation of Duryodhana though he was a king and had arranged a royal dinner for him, and went instead to Vidura, who was a low-born person and could only entertain Krishna as a poor man.

A strong and deep affection lives in our hearts for our son or father or wife; yet we go about our normal business and do not recite their names all the time. This is exactly how we should keep God in our minds and go on doing our duties at the same time.

Do your normal duty in service to God and worship of God. You can reach God through it. But if you think that your own duties are no good and take up other people's duties because they appeal to you better, you would lose your way and ruin yourself. Thus, doing your own duty and dedicating it to God is the golden rule to peace and happiness.

ALLAHABAD 1972
Introduction

During the Christmas holidays (1971) FCR had put together a number of recent sayings of the Shankaracharya in a form which he could learn by heart so as 'to hold the Universal Self (*Param-Atman*) in memory all the time'.

Having found great benefit from this practice, he issued these sayings to senior people in London and New York in the form of a 'New Year Programme' (1972).

At the same time a copy was sent to our interpreter (RLD) at the Ashram, who translated it into Hindi and read it to the Shankara-charya, who listened very attentively and sent his comments.

The Programme, and the reply (14 January) are here given together with a previous question (21 December 1971) and answer (also 14 January) on the same subject.

New Year Programme 1972
In desperation at my own inability to practise what I preach I recently found a shortcut which, so far, works well and is surprisingly simple. It could help anybody who desperately wants to take Step Two of the Ladder – Resolution – both those who have temporarily given up meditation or those who seem to be meditating happily, but deeply feel the need to take it further.

This programme can help the two half-hours, but does not take their place. It is meant for only a few people; if there is anyone you feel would benefit from its use, let me know.

We are given so many transient ideas that they pass us by, and we need just one to carry with us all the time. This 'shortcut' consists in committing to memory certain sentences from the Shankaracharya's recent talks designed to make us remember *Param-Atman* all the time – and in particular last thing at night and first thing in the morning.

We consist of an outer nervous system (cerebrospinal) through which we carry on our daily life, and a quite separate inner nervous system (autonomic). To achieve unity, we have to bring *both* together under the control of the causal level in the forebrain (Soul) and this is a good way to sow a seed there which can grow into a flowering shrub.

The method is to learn by heart a couplet, say, every week. This is most easily done by repeating with full attention the first sentence eight times, and then the second sentence eight times, and then both together eight times, so that the two are running in one's head to the exclusion of all other thoughts and desires before one goes to sleep; then one will wake up with them still in mind. There is no special order; choose whichever couplet appeals to you, continuing with it for some time until a change is needed.

Definition
Param-Atman is the *Atman* of the whole universe, living and non-living, conceivable and inconceivable.

Summary:
Vyasa, who wrote the *Bhagavad Gita*, says: 'I have made a critical study of all the scriptures (available to me) several times. The gist of all that, as I found, is that we should hold the *Param-Atman* (Universal Self) in memory all the time.'

Similarly, this single idea can include for us all other scriptures.

The first four couplets refer to the Inner life:

In the Soul (*Antahkarana*) of each person, there lives the universal (*Param-Atman*) along with the individual Self (*Jiva-Atman*) for the purpose of guidance.

Therefore we get a guiding Voice from time to time when we are in difficulties.

In order to hear that inner Voice, we should pray to the All-Knowing *Param-Atman* in solitude with a settled mind.

Then an answer, to bring us face to face with success, is sure to come forth.

Therefore what we have to do is to take guidance in our Soul from that immense source of energy, the *Param-Atman*, with fullest concentration of mind and in all humility.

This body (physical, subtle and causal) is the vehicle, and *Param-Atman* is the rider; regard the rider as separate from the vehicle.

Our mind has the property of thinking of something or other all the time; it cannot remain idle.

Thinking of *Param-Atman* leads to happiness, but thinking of worldly things leads only to unhappiness in the end.

The following four couplets can bring this same idea into one's daily activities in the outside world:

The states of consciousness which we experience are governed by the influx of *Sattva, Rajas* and *Tamas* in people, places, situations and events.
These all undergo change, but the Observer who sees them all as a passing show, always remains the same.

What to ordinary people are *different* shapes and forms are to a Realised person all manifestations of one and the same *Param-Atman*.
What he sees then, around and within himself, is *Param-Atman* and not the transient mirage which we call 'the world'.

Once you win over the *Param-Atman* by love, only then do you get all you need for a happy and profitable life.
But love is unconditional, and there is no place in the kingdom of love for demands and rewards.

A strong and deep affection lives in our own hearts for wife or son or parents, yet we go about our normal business without reciting their names all the time.
Each of us should try to serve the *Param-Atman* with that attribute in which we chiefly excel.

14 January
Answer to a letter from FCR dated 21 December 1971

HH: I have heard the thoughts expressed by you in your letter about the way you have adopted in order to remember *Param-*

Atman all the time. Your thoughts are highly commendable. The couplets you have selected[†] as a basis for further progress are very meaningful and unique in a way. Instead of saying anything else I would therefore send you only this message in token of my good wishes: that by going deeper and deeper into the source of your inner energy you are doing a great service to the uplift of your own Self and that of your circle.

3 January

Q: I find it comparatively easy to think about the *Param-Atman*, particularly in connection with the Laws of Nature in the universe and in man and in seeing that all that is going on in the outside world, whether it looks good or bad, is a part of One *Param-Atman*; but I would greatly appreciate help in developing a love or devotion to the *Param-Atman*, through what I suppose would be the practise of *Bhakti* (devotion). My capacity for love seems to be such a feeble thing and it is shown in the way I keep making demands upon you as our Teacher, instead of feeling for you as Shankaracharya and your wishes and living up to the Holy Tradition.

14 January
Reply from His Holiness

HH: You have asked for help in developing love or devotion to the *Param-Atman* through the practice of *Bhakti*, stating that your own capacity for love seems feeble. You should not worry on this account. Rather, you should know that the Path of Love is such

---

[†]New Year Programme 1972

26

a path that *Param-Atman* is pouring all His favours and blessings on it all the time. Love is not an action; it is a feeling. Love and True Knowledge are two names for one and the same thing, which is a natural manifestation of the *Atman* and it comes to the surface automatically when the *Antahkarana* concentrates. Then you get the 'feel' of it.

Through your beneficial and holy efforts, let your own fullness see the fullness of the *Param-Atman*, and let the practice, the practitioner and the object of practice merge together to form one single identity. Then the world as such disappears and the *Param-Atman* appears in its place. This summarises the philosophy of *Bhakti* through love.

13 January
Mela Talk

The previous speaker spoke about the fear of death, which haunts the minds of even the bravest people.

His Holiness picked up the same theme. He said that everybody fears death – whether great or small, learned or ignorant, but there is no such thing as death. The so-called 'death' is nothing but a natural corollary of the phenomenon of birth. The only way to avoid death is to avoid being born. It is not possible to be born and not to die.

Actually the individual Self, living in the body, is immortal. It gives up an old body in order to put on a new body, just as we give up our old clothes and put on new ones. If we are happy to discard an old garment and put on a new one, there is no reason to be unhappy when the Self discards an old body and adopts a new one.

> An Indian went to Africa. When his money was finished he went to a moneylender to ask for a loan. Just then, there was a death in an Indian family living in that neighbourhood and the people of the family were weeping. The moneylender asked the Indian why his countrymen living in that house were weeping. He replied that it was a custom in his country to weep when there is a death in the family.
>
> The moneylender asked again, 'And what do you do when there is a birth in the family?' The Indian said, 'Then we rejoice.'
>
> The moneylender said, 'Then, if you are the sort of person who rejoices when receiving a thing but weeps when you have to return it, I certainly won't lend *you* any money!'

A person who has died has never written back to say what happened to him after death. Therefore, the only course open to us is to take authority from our Holy Scriptures on the subjects relating to death and thereafter. We can find a lot of information there on these subjects. The following teachings from the *Bhagavad Gita* tell us how to deal with death:

> Forget the past. Do not fear for the future either. Devote the *present* to the *Bhakti* of the *Param-Atman*. A devotee of the *Param-Atman* never perishes.

> For two half-hours a day, give up all duties and obligations; surrender yourself completely to the single

care and protection of the *Param-Atman*. He will save
you from all evil consequences, and therein would lie the
end of all your worries.

One who sees *Param-Atman* in everybody and everything,
and sees everybody and everything in *Param-Atman*,
Param-Atman never becomes obscure to him and he
never becomes obscure to *Param-Atman*.

We fear death because, under the influence of *Maya*, we have
forgotten ourSelves. And it is this forgetting of the Divine Self
which makes for us all the troubles we get. It is not God who is
the maker of our troubles.

16 January
Mela Talk

His Holiness referred to the story of Shri Sukadeva, the son of
the famous author of ancient times, Shri Vyasa.

Shri Sukadeva was a child prodigy who had already
attained Self Realisation. So, as soon as he could, he
started running towards the jungles.

But he was the only child of Vyasa, born to him in his
old age, after he had waited for issue all his life. Seeing
him thus running away, Vyasa was grief-stricken and he
ran after him crying, 'My son! My son! Come back!'

But Sukadeva went ahead without looking back. A
river lay on his way. Some women were bathing in it
undressed. They saw Sukadeva passing close to them, but
they did not pay any heed to him and continued to enjoy
their nude bathing. Subsequently Vyasa also reached

29

them pursuing Sukadeva. But on seeing him, the women hid themselves behind the trees and hurriedly put on their clothes.

Vyasa asked them why they did not mind the presence of his young son when they were naked, and why clothes became necessary before an old man like him. The women replied, 'Your son saw his own Self in us. You are old, but the sexual hangover, which responds to the difference between a man and a woman, still continues to affect your vision.'

Thus, if we see differences in worldly things – 'this is this, that is that' – instead of seeing everything as part of our own Self, then there will be things which we like and also things which we dislike. These likes and dislikes lead to unhappiness.

A person who practises *Bhakti*, uses his speech for expressing the properties of *Param-Atman*, and his eye for seeing Him everywhere. He is reluctant to use organs otherwise.

In this way he is practising *Bhakti* everywhere, whether he is in a jungle or at his house. You are listening to this talk about the *Param-Atman*. This is also *Bhakti*. But no action, by itself, is *Bhakti*. Cover every act with the thought of *Bhakti*, and every act becomes an act of *Bhakti*. Thus growing crops on a field, sitting at a shop selling things, and all such things, can be converted into *Bhakti* if they are done with a spirit of service to the *Param-Atman*.

Bhakti is a power of the heart. Let this single power of *Bhakti* drive all your actions, just as a single electric main drives all the machinery in a factory.

When we give up the world in quest of *Bhakti*, the giving up should be mental also, and not merely physical. A physical sort of giving up, without a corresponding mental attitude and the mind still harbouring desires, is hypocrisy. It does not contribute to happiness.

In the mind of a busy householder, the idea of *Bhakti* is sometimes lost sight of in the midst of daily engagements. The way to reverse it is to read holy works like the *Bhagavad-Gita* (or the Gospels). This should be done as a daily routine by anyone who wants to practise *Bhakti*.

> A rich man used to go to a Mahatma, but he used to talk to him about his household affairs only. The Mahatma asked him the reason, and he replied that it was because his household people loved him very much. Therefore they were always uppermost in his mind. The Mahatma went to his house one day and gave a sewing needle to his wife. He said to her, 'Your husband seems to be planning to take all his things with him when he goes into the next world. Tell him to carry this needle also (if he can) for my sake. I shall need it there for sewing my torn clothes.' When she told this to her husband, he understood the truth about worldly belongings.

So, you should try to hoard that which you *can* take with you, that is, *Bhakti*, and not that which would be left here, that is, the worldly possessions. Transfer your attachment to *Param-Atman*. This is *Bhakti*. Under the influence of *Bhakti*, everything undergoes a transformation. Poverty becomes riches, poison becomes nectar. There is pain and suffering in the world only as long as faith in *Param-Atman* is not there.

20 January
Mela Talk

Some 1½ to 2 million devotees have had their dip in the holy waters of the Ganges, and earned a profit. A trader is happy when there is a profit. But what about a loss?

In this 'trade' of life, all of us want a profit and want to avoid a loss. The first two verses of the *Isha Upanishad* tell us the way. They say:

> The entire living and non-living world constituting this universe should be taken as covered by one single *Param-Atman*, that is, as a manifestation of one single *Param-Atman*. Make your living in this world with the things thus provided to you, without desiring money from anyone else. But *Param-Atman* does not assert His ownership over what He gives to the world (like air, water, food, etc,). Similarly, while using them for your living, you should not consider them as belonging to you or yourself to be the owner.

> Desire a hundred-year-long life thus lived, and full of action. There is no other way to avoid a coating of evil while leading a human life.

According to the *Bhagavad Gita*, Arjuna refused to fight the war of *Mahabharata* and Krishna persuaded him to do so. He explained to him that even in case he does not heed his advice, his own nature and temperament would force him into battle. In this way our nature, habits and tendencies compel us into good and bad actions. Therefore we should try to change the evil tendencies in our nature to better ones.

People often complain that although they have been practising *Bhakti* or meditation over a number of years, they do not appear to be deriving any benefit from it. This is because their tendencies and nature have not changed.

We should bear in mind that whatever the Creator has given to the world, He has 'given it up' to the world. He no longer asserts any ownership over it. We also should cultivate the habit of using and enjoying it as His gift and not our own property. This attitude will correct our evil tendencies, and then the practice of *Bhakti* or meditation will begin bearing fruit.

It is not gold or worldly possessions which are evil, only identification with them.

Once four men set out on a business trip, carrying firearms for protection. They met a Mahatma on their road. He warned them not to go that way as there was danger ahead. They did not listen to him and said that they were well equipped to face any threat. As they went further, they found a gold ingot lying on the ground. Rejoicing at their find, they wrapped it up in a piece of cloth with the idea of dividing it among themselves.

As night fell, two of them went to a neighbouring village to get some food, two staying behind. When they had gone, those staying behind felt tempted to keep the ingot for themselves and conspired to shoot the other two when they returned with food.

At the same time, those who had gone to the village had a hearty meal in an eating shop. While returning with food for the other two, they also succumbed to the temptation of keeping the gold ingot for themselves and conspired to do away with the other two. Therefore they mixed poison with the food they were taking for them. When they returned with the food, the other two shot them dead. But being hungry, they at once devoured the food brought for them. They fell asleep, never to wake again.

Next morning the same Mahatma passed there on his way to the river for his daily bath. He found the four lying dead, and the gold ingot wrapped in the cloth. He threw it into the river so that it might not do further mischief.

This is how we meet mishaps in our daily life owing to our reasoning being polluted by evil tendencies. If we consider and use everything as a gift from the *Param-Atman*, and thus practise *Bhakti*, then our reasoning becomes clear and we can lead a long and happy life as expressed in those *Upanishad* verses.

Evil associations cause evil tendencies in our reasoning, and they, in turn, result in evil actions. Good associations cause good tendencies and result in good actions. We should all try to achieve a hundred-year-long life, full of happiness and useful action by following this teaching of the *Upanishad*. Such a life would be a good worldly life, good for us and good for the world.

Once I had occasion to address a meeting of prominent scientists in Delhi. I found a slogan displayed there reading: 'We search for light in the darkness.' I liked the theme and devoted my address to that subject. We also look for light in the darkness. But the sun's light fails to show up the world. When mind gets still, a true light shines and we see the world in its true colours.

23 January
Mela Talk

In the ageless continuum of time, it seems so futile to take account of all the events that go on making and unmaking themselves in an unending chain. A little while ago we were preparing to set up this *Mela*. Now we are preparing to wind it up. Thus anything that begins has to end, and anybody who comes into the world has to go.

Many people say there is no rebirth. Actually, each birth writes down the destiny of death, and each death writes down the destiny of birth. The *Gita* says that there is neither any 'birth' nor any 'death', but it is merely a change that is going on all the time. One who sees a changelessness in all the changes that are going on, sees correctly.

It is a body that is born and dies. The *Atman* Himself, who inhabits the body, is birthless and deathless. *It is enough to understand only this much of the subject, because in trying to understand everything we often end by understanding nothing at all.*

The *Param-Atman* also incarnates but, unlike ordinary people, His incarnation is Divine. Why His birth is Divine and that of ordinary people not divine, is due to *associations*. Two examples will illustrate the difference between the two:

> An ordinary person, on joining state service, had to sign an undertaking that he would do his work honestly and impartially. On the wall of many offices a picture of Mahatma Ghandi is displayed with one hand holding a walking stick, and the other hand with its five fingers

raised in the gesture of blessing people. But dishonest people point towards this picture and say, 'Look! Ghandi is showing five fingers to indicate that a one rupee bribe is not enough. Let it be five at least!'

Such would be the behaviour of an ordinary person. Now we will consider a Divine Incarnation:

The child Krishna once wanted to go out grazing cows along with the other boys. Everybody tried to dissuade him for he was too young to remain out the whole day, but he insisted on going. Yashoda, his mother, then gave some boiled sweets to the boys and asked them to give them to him when he felt hungry, to save him from the hot sun, fatigue etc. Then the boys and Krishna went to the bank of the river Yamuna to graze the cows. There, Krishna appeared to be eating the sand of the Yamuna instead of the sweets, and when told not to indulge in such a dirty habit he did not stop.

In the evening, when they returned to the village, they complained to Mother Yashoda about Krishna's mischievous behaviour. She questioned Krishna, and he denied it point-blank.

Then she caught Krishna with one hand, took up a stick with the other, and threatened to beat him. Krishna said, 'Mother, just peep into my mouth. If I ate sand, you will surely see it there.'

Yashoda looked into Krishna's mouth. First she saw only his lovely pinkish lips and pearly white teeth. But soon she began seeing in it the whole village – their own house – another Yashoda holding another Krishna – another earth and another sky – mountains and rivers –

and the whole universe. She was completely nonplussed. Seeing her frightened out of her wits, Krishna withdrew the vision and assumed his former appearance.

This is an example of a Divine Incarnation.

Letter of 6 April

Why the incarnation of *Param-Atman* is Divine, but that of ordinary people not divine, is due to association:

Param-Atman incarnates of His own free will. Ordinary people are reborn as a consequence of their own actions.

Param-Atman incarnates to attract people towards Him and for their own good. An ordinary person is reborn to reap what he has sowed.

Param-Atman incarnates with the *Maya* under His full control. An ordinary person is under the control of *Maya* all the time.

Param-Atman is not bound by the results of His actions. An ordinary person is bound.

Param-Atman is beyond pleasure and pain. An ordinary person is not so.

Pain is inevitable for embodied beings, but one could be free from *suffering* if one gives up attachment.

We should not try to renounce suffering, but to bear it. If we take a debt, we should repay it rather than renounce it.

Mela Talk continued

In order to recognise and experience Divine manifestations, a devotee has to renounce everything else. By renouncing every-thing he comes to possess everything. Another story illustrates this.

> A Mahatma, Swami Vishuddhananda, was living in the Himalayas. The Maharaja of Tehri, then a Himalayan state, was greatly devoted to him. One day he asked the Mahatma, 'Master, what are the indications of a person who has renounced the world?'
>
> The Mahatma kicked him out of the cottage saying, 'Get out. Carrying all the dirt of the world on you as you do, you have no business to ask questions about the indications of a renounced person.'
>
> The Maharaja departed, but stayed outside the cottage the whole night. At three o'clock in the morning the Mahatma chanced to come out and asked, 'Who is sitting there?'
>
> 'The one whom you kicked out', said the Maharaja.
>
> 'Do you see the indication of a renounced person now?', said the Mahatma. 'He is entirely fearless, so that he can kick out even a Maharaja.'

Since a fully Realised person renounces everything, people think that he must be undergoing great suffering since he may be without even the bare necessities of life. But he does not feel any sufferings. He feels all the comforts of heaven with the little he has got or even nothing at all. *Pain and suffering are two different things.* Pain is a bodily experience while suffering is mental. All embodied beings must be subject to physical pain. The *Atman* however, sees the pleasures and pains of the body but is not subject to either. Pleasures and physical comforts are meant for those to whom worldly enjoyment is the be-all and end-all of life. A *Bhakta* (devotee) cares little for them.

If we run after the pleasures of the physical senses, the advantage of being born human is missed. Animals and birds also eat, drink, build nests, reproduce, look after their offspring, etc. But the advantage of a human body is that you can open your inner eye and see your real Self. Birds and animals cannot do this.

The ancient books say that there are eighty-four thousand million kinds of living beings, and a being (*Jiva*) goes on wandering from one form of life to another till *Param-Atman*, out of pity for its sheer misery, gives it the body of a man. If you fulfil the purpose of having a human body in this life, then you have made a success of it. Your visit to the *Mela* is meant for this purpose only.

22 April
Comment on Mela Talk 23 January
Divine Incarnation

HH: The incarnations of *Param-Atman* are such that they have powers to alter the whole course of events and of Nature even. Thus they can only be rare like Lord Krishna, etc. They may be total or partial.

When He reveals Himself in the *Antahkarana* of a *Bhakta*, it is a case of revelation rather than of incarnation. But it might also be called a partial incarnation, in a restricted sense. Such cases, however, should be carefully discriminated from mere hallucinations in weak minds.

29 January
Mela Talk

This body is like a big town – the habitation of many. It contains a whole world of living creatures inside. They all possess life and desire to live. Some appear harmful and some useful. They are constantly being kept in a state of dynamic equilibrium, and this equilibrium keeps the body fit. Any disturbance of equilibrium causes disease; then compensating forces of nature arise which tend to set it right. Similarly, when the balance in creation is upset, then the forces of *Param-Atman* come into play to restore it.

Nature is constantly striving for perfection, never attaining it. Man also, as part of Nature. One who is ill tries to get well, one who is weak tries to get strong, one who is poor tries to get rich, and so on. Thus, in every situation, there is dissatisfaction, and there are corresponding efforts to overcome it and to improve things.

But the more we try to improve, the worse everything seems to get. We say we have progressed, but we also say that the olden days were golden days. Similarly, today, which seems full of causes for dissatisfaction, will tomorrow become a golden day. Gandhi in his time considered taxation to be excessive and launched agitation against it. But the taxation of those days is now considered very light compared with today's.

The reason is that increase of material facilities do not contribute to happiness; instead it is *taking a rational attitude* that promotes happiness. If our planning is good, then even fewer facilities would be enough to create happiness.

Our efforts, however, are more towards *looking* good externally and less towards *being* so internally. Trying to look good outside, but staying bad inside, is wilful deception. Such attempts can only result in harm.

> Once a well-dressed young man came to me and posed
> as a son of the Prince of Avagarh. He said that he was
> stranded at the railway station as he had lost all his
> luggage, and he wanted a loan, promising to return it by
> telegraphic money order as soon as he got home. I told
> him to first make himself comfortable at the Ashram
> and have his meal, and that we would consider later
> what we could do about it. By chance, an employee of
> Avagarh State also happened to be in the Ashram at that
> time. I asked him if he knew the man and he denied all
> knowledge of him. The imposter then disappeared on
> some pretext and never returned.

The world, on the whole, is like this. People put on good appearances outside and keep ulterior motives within.

Trying to do good to our own fellow beings is the first thing to do. One who does not serve his fellow beings is far from serving the *Param-Atman*. The *Param-Atman* gives us a decent human body at the time of our birth. But, by the time it is taken back, we have polluted it by all sorts of unholy actions, done during our lifetime. In this connection the saint and poet Kabir has said: 'Everyone was given a shawl (the human body) to cover himself with, but all made it dirty during use. But Kabir also used it, and doing so carefully, he returned it neat and clean.'

29 March
Extract from a letter to Dr DC from RL Dixit
Answer to an enquiry about the orange-coloured robes worn by
Mahatmas – whether this colour attracted Sattva.

The question made His Holiness smile, and he said, 'Yes, it
attracts Sattva.' Orange, and more precisely, yellow, is the colour
worn by Lord Vishnu. Devotees also wear this colour for its
purifying effect on the mind.

However, sannyasins who have renounced the world wear a
hematite colour which contains a greater proportion of red than
orange. This is because it is the colour of fire. Fire burns all
worldly things whether good or bad. Not only that, but it also
changes everything into its own shape – fire – and fire is a great
purifier. Similarly, a renounced person burns all his worldly
impulses whether good or bad, transforming them all into his
own, pure Self. The fire in this case is True Knowledge. This fire
of True Knowledge burns away the entire false illusion of the
world, 'this is good, this is bad', and all that is left subsequently
is pure Reality.

The wearing of the orange or the hematite colour is meant to
remind the wearer constantly of his duty, just as wearing a
uniform reminds a policeman or soldier of his duty.

4 April
Discourse
Context. Chapter 8, verse 3 of the *Bhagavad Gita:*

'He who frees himself of his body remembering *Param-Atman* at
his last moment, gets into *Param-Atman* undoubtedly.'

The Holy Scriptures lay down that at all times – in the beginning, in the middle, and in the end – all of the past, the present and the future – one should always think of *Param-Atman*, because we do not know when the end may come. But we cannot do this without forming a habit. However, it is wrong to imagine, as some people do, that they could form this habit in their old age. If we do not cultivate this habit in our younger days, it is difficult to do so when we are old. But even if you do manage only to remember *Param-Atman* in old age, and not when you were young, He would be satisfied even then!

This world wants your body. Well, serve the world with your body. But *Param-Atman* wants your love only. If you love *Param-Atman* it would be *Param-Atman* who would then begin to serve you. The *Bhagavad Gita* says:

> Through the inner ear of a *Bhakta* (devotee), I make my way into his *Antahkarana* and sweep it clean.

Facilities and conveniences increase desires, ultimately creating unrest. Therefore *Param-Atman* takes away the facilities from a *Bhakta* and he becomes a poor man.

A Mahatma lived in the jungle, and his hut was so small that it could accommodate only three persons. Once a severe storm with heavy rain came. A lone traveller stood outside the hut, exposed to wind and rain. The Mahatma called him in and asked him to sit down. Then a second man came and he was also called in.

Then a third man came who was rather bulky. Now all had to stand up since there was no room for four people to sit there. This third man was rich and he offered to build a big room in place of the small hut, so that many people could sit in it.

The Mahatma drove them all out saying, 'You want to demolish the hut which gave you shelter. I do not want your bigger room for it would only increase the crowd around me, distract me from my work, and increase my desires.'

Facilities lead to desires, and desires mean death.

There are troubles on every path. So the path of *Bhakti* (Devotion) also has its own troubles; but these troubles carry us forward and form the basis of fresh uplift. By bearing these troubles the *Bhakti* strengthens, we form the habit of constantly remembering *Param-Atman*, and are thus able to remember *Param-Atman* at the time of death. A *Bhakta* is desireless and peaceful. He has no enmity. His vision is uniform. He sees *Param-Atman* in everything.

A good housewife serves well all the guests that come to her house. But she does so only out of her regard for her husband. Similarly we should serve everybody, but out of our regard for *Param-Atman*.

Radha meditated on Krishna, and Krishna meditated on Radha. As this meditation deepened, Radha turned into Krishna and Krishna turned into Radha. These transformations from one to the other took place every instant, until the difference between the two vanished.

Similarly, through the deepening of *Bhakti* (love) the difference between *Bhakta* (devotee) and *Param-Atman* vanishes and it is no longer possible to differentiate which is which.

Therefore, thinking of *Param-Atman*, we should be able to stop worrying about the world – at first for half an hour, but later for always.

15 April
Ashram Talk

Poverty Blissful
Poverty is bliss because if *Bhakti* develops in it, the image of *Param-Atman* begins to live in the *Antahkarana* just as the image of an object lives in a mirror. And a man thus possessing the image of the Almighty in his heart could no longer be called poor. But a poor man who entertains desires is certainly miserable, while a poor man with no desires at all is happy.

Alesko
In olden times there lived in China a man called Alesko. He kept nothing with him except a piece of gunny (sackcloth) to wrap around his body. The king needed a person to manage the affairs of his kingdom who had no personal ambitions. When he heard about Alesko he wanted to try him and sent his men to call him. They found him playing with turtles in a pool of mud.

'Lucky man', they said, 'your days of poverty are over. His Majesty, the King, has summoned you to appoint you his Prime Minister.'

Alesko said, 'Is it true that His Majesty keeps a turtle wrapped in a sheet of gold and worships it every day?'

'Yes, it is true.'

'Is that turtle alive or dead?' 'It is dead of course.'

'Would any of the turtles you see here like to be kept like that as long as it is alive?' 'No.'

'If even an animal would not give up his natural surroundings for being kept in gold, how do you expect me to do so? That turtle is dead, as you say.

Similarly, I also can surrender my liberty only when I am dead.'

Succumbing to flattery in order to escape poverty is to kill one's own life.

Doing One's Duty.
Where the *Bhagavad Gita* prescribes 'giving up' it also explains how to give up. What we have to give up is the desire to derive benefit from our actions – and not actions themselves. If we give up acting but continue to indulge in desires, then we would simply be pretending to give up. Before undertaking an action, an ordinary worldly man always tries to assess what benefit would accrue to him as a result of that action. But a Realised man undertakes it as a matter of duty, with no desire for its consequential benefits.

Guru Deva and Language
When the preceding Shankaracharya went to Lucknow, people told him that the town possessed an Urdu culture and spoke Urdu language. He replied that it would not matter. He would do his duty irrespective of the extent of the benefit people derived from his visit.

Before trying to do good to others, we should first try to improve our own selves. We cannot save a drowning man if we cannot swim ourselves.

Correct attitudes make real wealth. One who possesses this wealth is never poor.

17 April
Questions from Mrs S

What is it that divides the physical from the subtle, the subtle from the causal, and all those three from Pure Consciousness itself? Is it energy? Is it thought in the subtle body? Does everyone have a physical, subtle and causal body? If the energy of matter in a chair is raised, does it become subtle? What is the difference between matter and consciousness? What has all this got to do with Self-realisation?

Regarding the three worlds we live in, I have often wondered about the difference between the physical and subtle worlds. The other day I tried out a recipe. I found that at every step of making the dish, it was not going as it was meant to. Could I take it that the recipe was in the subtle world and the act of cooking was in the physical world? It just struck me at that time how easy it was mentally and how different it was physically!

2 May
Reply from His Holiness

His Holiness says that physical, subtle and causal are just three states in which a being lives. The dividing line between them exists as a natural phenomenon but it is not energy. Thought is in *Buddhi*. Everyone has a physical, subtle and causal body.

The question about raising the energy of a chair is too hypothetical as the three states are not interchangeable.

The difference between matter and consciousness is that of cause and effect. The object of knowing all this is that it is helpful in attaining Self-realisation.

The making of the dish was not going as it was meant to because the *Buddhi* was not helping enough.

Apart from *Buddhi*, the factor of *Prarabdha*[†] also comes in with regard to success in doing a thing. If *Buddhi* and *Prarabdha* both support a physical act, things go as desired and success is inevitable.

9 May
Question from FCR

I must know something of the meaning of the word '*Prarabdha*' which I have never heard before. If you cannot find an equivalent English word, could you give me some small description or example of its use?

Answer from D
I could not find an exactly equivalent English word for the Sanskrit word '*Prarabdha*' used by His Holiness, and I did not attempt to explain it as you had told me once that you already had a good Sanskrit-English dictionary in your library which I

[†]See also next question and answer and page 101.

thought might explain it better than I could. It belongs to the concept of rebirth and as such, it might make no sense to those who do not believe in any such phenomenon.

Out of the many countless good and bad acts done by an individual in all his past lives, *Prarabdha* is that parcel of them, for reaping the consequences of which his present life is intended. It is an extraneous factor to govern our life, in addition to what we do now, which is called '*Purushartha*'. *Purushartha* and *Prarabdha* going together make for success in an enterprise. *Prarabdha* is inescapable and it would search us out wherever we may be, just as a calf can search out its mother from among a hundred cows. It manifests itself as what we call 'luck' or 'chance' or 'destiny', etc.

Further Question from FCR

Recently, I once more told the story of the parrot and his master, the intellectual man, who did not put his teacher's instructions into practice. Following this, I tried to carry out certain of His Holiness's instructions to me. Next morning, I woke up with a clear and happy feeling as if I saw the whole of my ego or personality, like that of the intellectual, as from the point of view of the liberated parrot sitting in the tree! I still have the feeling and keep noticing that there is an incessant commentary going on in the mind about what one sees – approving, disapproving, etc. Is not this a useless part of the mind which could be made to observe impartially like an interpreter?

HH: The incessant commentary going on in the mind about what one sees – approving, disapproving, etc, is certainly a useless part of the mind. One method to avoid it is to observe impartially, considering yourself as separate from the mind, as you yourself said. The other method is to make the mind engage in good thoughts only, so that it gets no opportunity to entertain wrong ideas. This amounts to keeping the mind under control as you would a servant. Let your mind be the servant and you its master.

17 April
Ashram Talk

The *Brahma Sutra* of the *Vedas* has ten entirely different commentaries to explain what is *Param-Atman* and what is not *Param-Atman*. One school of thought considers the *Atman* as the ultimate Reality; another says it is *Shakti* (power), which is so; and yet another that the ultimate Reality is absolutely void – a total absence of everything. Some say there is nothing except *Param-Atman*, while others say there must be two – the *Param-Atman* and the *Jiva-Atman*. No two sages have spoken alike. Chaitanya Mahaprabhu propounded the doctrine of *Kirtan*, while Shankaracharya pleaded for *Advaita* (there is nothing but *Param-Atman*). Thus one feels lost in a jungle of diverse opinions and wonders what to do. The solution is to follow the example of great men and, like them, obtain Realisation for oneself.

There are endless suppositions about the world and about *Param-Atman*. These relate to the practical life as well as to spiritual life. Shankaracharya has accepted both.

All of these diversities of thought are recognised only in the verses of the *Vedas*. They recognise the infinite, formless *Param-Atman* as well as the finite personified *Param-Atman*. Hence the *Vedas* are a complete repository of all ideas, accommodating all shades of opinion and leaving out nothing.

> A monkey sat on the roof of a railway carriage, and when a passenger put his head out of a window, the monkey quietly descended, pinched his cap and climbed back on to the roof. The bystanders advised the passenger to give the monkey something to eat in order to get his cap back. When he passed up a banana, the monkey held the banana in one hand but hung on to the cap with the other. When offered a second banana, the monkey took it but dropped the cap on the railway line where it was irretrievably lost!

We are all temperamentally greedy like the monkey, and there are innumerable temptations in the world to attract our greed. The force of these attractions is irresistible, and we continue to fall victim to them all the time. These forces are desires – sex, anger, attachment, greed, vanity, jealousy – which keep beguiling us and from which we find it difficult to escape. The only escape lies in renunciation. It looks difficult, but it comes with practice. Just practise transferring your love of these attractions to *Param-Atman*.

Attachment to worldly things is the root cause of all our troubles. But we little realise that it is all false, and that we are bound to get deceived if we take worldly things seriously. All hopes are false. Once your mind gets set in love for *Param-Atman*, the world would cease to attract you.

> Somebody was feeding a Mahatma. He asked the Mahatma, 'How do you like the taste of this food?' The Mahatma replied, 'I feel as if I am not eating at all.'

It is the body that eats, while we feel that we eat. This is a delusion. It is the engine that takes the fuel, not the driver. And the food taken differs from case to case. A baby's food is milk and an adult's food is grain, a snake's food is rats, and so on. Just as the body's nourishment is food and water, similarly *Manas's* nourishment is holy intention, *Buddhi's* is thought, *Atman's* is joy, nourishment for bodily organs is legitimate gratification. Giving this nourishment to each in proper doses is leading a controlled life. The advantage of a controlled life is that it would be what you want it to be.

5 May
Question from CL to His Holiness

Even if one read all the wonderful descriptions which the Shankaracharya has given us of the *Param-Atman*; even if one read everything that the great teachers of the past have written too; even then, surely, one would be left with one's own interpretation of their words, one's own concepts and mental images of what *Param-Atman* is like?

But if through the meditation, one were to reach that place within one where the *Param-Atman* dwells, is it not true to say that one would have direct experience of His being instead of inventing thoughts and concepts, one would directly *be* what the *Param-Atman* is? And would not this direct experience of His being come to one through the sound of the Mantra, so that at any time during the day or night the repetition of this sound would bring it back again?

16 May
Reply from His Holiness

It is true to say that one would have direct experience of His being if one were to reach, through meditation, that place within one where *Param-Atman* dwells. It is also true that a direct experience of His being would come through the sound of the Mantra.

Regarding the varying thoughts and concepts, in the beginning we have to accept them in order to get over them later on. As one passes through them and goes ahead with the help of one's own power of reasoning and understanding, only then a final stage is reached where a confusion of ideas ceases, otherwise not. For example, the *Upanishad* says that after realising *Param-Atman* the Holy Scriptures are useless, and they are also useless if we do not realise *Param-Atman*. However, their purpose is to increase our interest in meditation, to promote our zeal in attaining our object, and to make us more and more capable of experiencing and realising.

8 August
Reply from D to FCR's letter giving story of a London tramp apropos the remark by the Shankaracharya that the subtle level often creates dreams out of unfulfilled desires and fears experienced by the individual, thereby working them out of a person's system:

What you have just read made me think of a story about a tramp who slept in Hyde Park and was happy because he always dreamt he was sleeping in the Ritz Hotel. Someone who was interested in him booked him a room for the night in the Ritz. Next morning they asked him how he had slept. 'Very badly', he replied, 'I spent the night dreaming I was sleeping on a hard bench in the park!'

HH liked it and spoke on that subject at some length. The substance of what he said is:

The story is very useful in understanding the working of the human mind. It is never satisfied with what it has, and always desires the opposite. While a poor man envies the comforts of the rich and wants to be rich too, a rich man is weary of his anxieties and envies the carefree sleep of one who has nothing. A sick man worries about getting well (only making his sickness worse), while a man in good health worries that he may get ill.

The mind also has a tendency to live more in the past and the future, and less in the present which is much more important than either. This combination of dissatisfaction with the present and the perpetual desire for the opposite in the future causes perpetual unhappiness. *The remedy is to see, with the eye of True Knowledge, the same thing in everything*, and that same thing is *Param-Atman*. Then the outlook becomes balanced and unified, unrest giving place to tranquillity.

However, in our day-to-day actions (on the physical level), as apart from our thoughts, things should be taken as they are, and not everything as the same.

7 September
Reply to letter from FCR of 17 August

You have asked what word His Holiness used for 'mind' when he was commenting on the dreams of the London tramp, whether it was *Manas* or *Buddhi*. He used *Manas*. *Buddhi* is used in a different context.

8 August

The following question was sent by Mr Rabeneck direct to Interpreter Dixit, and answered by His Holiness:

Q: When looking at the street, buildings and people under a changing sky, or at clouds and trees, there comes a feeling of all this being moved by *Param-Atman*. Such a unity in my perception may last for about half-an-hour.

When complete silence comes in meditation there is a vague feeling of an expanding and dissolving flow, there is unity for several minutes.

But in life there is no feeling that events in which 'I' am involved are a 'passing show'. An obstinate sense of separateness and of being the 'doer' remains. Is 'keeping the *Param-Atman* in mind as much as possible' all one has to do, or should there be more order and discipline introduced on physical and subtle levels, and how?

HH: When looking at the street, buildings and people under a changing sky, or at clouds and trees – and also when there is a vague feeling of an expanding and dissolving flow – what you experience is the WORLD. And the world has three stages: creation, maintenance and destruction.

When we wake up from sleep, the (sensory) world stands up before us as it is; when we perceive a dream, however, it is a dreamworld that we see. When we go into deep and dreamless sleep, then everything of the world merges into the Self, and only that Self is all in all. That is why we try to merge everything into our own Self in our day-to-day life.

The advantage of this would be that the thought of the past and of the future would weaken and you would find yourself in a special stage of Self-consciousness. As this practice deepens, you would see the states of waking and dreaming more and more alike. With your eyes open or shut, it would be the same world before you. A condition of sameness would possess your heart. The mind (*Manas*) would shed its burden and become filled with joy instead. A feeling of perfection and limitlessness would supervene.

In sending us this question and answer Mr R wrote:

'You will see yourself from the enclosed copy how fully and clearly he has answered my first question. And then he describes the further steps, what to expect and what to aim for. In fact, it is a programme of work for a long time to come.'

ALLAHABAD 1972
First Audience
Tuesday 3 October

After greetings had been exchanged, and the proposal accepted that each of us (RA, MA, JR, FCR) should put our own questions in turn, the Shankaracharya remarked:

HH: It is worthwhile to catch some of the spiritual influences which are available here. Although practically everything has been discussed before in our talks, it is so very nice to be together and to refresh the memory once again and see each other.

Question from JR
I would like to thank His Holiness for allowing me to come and I would like to ask him how to improve the quality of my meditation, as I feel this would be a way to increase my capacity of love for the *Param-Atman*.

HH: Although individuals do feel a separate identity, in reality there is only one identity, and that is the *Param-Atman*. In our *Antahkarana*, the inner body, and the subtle body, we have this individual being, and because of ignorance and other influences, it seems to feel a difference from the *Param-Atman*, and that is why it wants to unite with the *Param-Atman*. For this unity of the individual and the Universal it seems as if the effort is being made by the individual himself. The individual, if indeed he does anything at all, only removes the impediments which block his vision of the unity of the *Param-Atman*. In fact, the movement is only from the *Param-Atman*'s side. It is *Param-Atman* who reaches out to the individual Himself. The love or devotion should be

57

developed by removing the impediments and that, of course, is possible through the meditation and the attention which one brings into one's life; and this, in a way, removes the identity of the individual which is composed of his name, his form and his so-called being. All these things have got to be given up for the real Unity or for the real Love towards the *Param-Atman*. The effort is, of course, made by the individual, but he makes little effort. The greater effort is made by the *Param-Atman*. Just as a small being or child has small legs, so he can walk only a few steps, the big man can walk quicker and cover more ground. The same applies to the individual, who is a very small being, and the *Param-Atman* which has no limit. This is how the unity of the individual and the *Param-Atman* should be made.

All individuals are the Absolute themselves, and so are you. It is only a question of realising that one is the Absolute. To realise *that* one has to do away with these impediments, and to illustrate this, there is a story of a lion cub:

> Once, in the forest, a lioness who had several cubs went off to search for food, and while she was away one of the cubs strayed and got into the middle of a flock of sheep. The cub followed the sheep, and the shepherd, seeing the cub with the sheep, kept him. The cub behaved like the sheep because of the company of the sheep. The shepherd thought that if he remained in this forest, then one day the lioness would roar and the cub, hearing the roar, would remember it was a lion and would attack the sheep. So he took the flock with the cub to another forest where he believed there were no lions.
>
> One day, a lion *did* roar in this other forest. All the sheep ran away, and the cub also tried to run away.

The lion asked the cub to stop and said, 'Why are you afraid of me? There is no need, you are not a sheep, you are a lion like me. If you are not sure I can show you.' So he took him to a pond and the little lion saw in the reflection that he had the same face and same characteristics as the one who roared. Then the lion asked him to roar with him. So he learnt how to roar, and the whole personality and individuality of this little lion was completely changed. He started roaring like a lion.

All our efforts in the world are learning the language of the world, which is like the language of the sheep and the life of the sheep. By good company – the company of saints – and through discourses, we learn to give up the language of the world and take to the language of the spirit. Once we have learnt, and have seen how saintly persons who are nearer the Absolute conduct their lives – we also can be like this young lion and start behaving like a proper lion, because we are all proper lions by nature.

Question from MA

The remembrance of *Param-Atman* during the day is an increasing comfort and nowadays everything is more pleasant, and even unpleasant things seem less important than before. However, one feels on a dreamy plateau where, because of the pleasant life, the *need* to keep moving on the path is less sharp. One is not complaining about the increased happiness, but though one feels the greater presence during the day, one's meditation does not seem deep enough and one seems more caught in a dreamy phase. Can His Holiness advise?

HH: One of the fundamental characteristics of life on this earth is the worldly illusion of being the independent doer, of having free will. It is very difficult to maintain that individuals are the doers of anything, for the whole creation is a manifestation of the Absolute who is the real doer. He has made His whole show in such a beautiful pattern that it keeps changing from one moment to another, and must keep on multiplying also. The whole thing is going on by virtue of the creative impulse given by the Absolute; He is the independent one, He is the free one, and He is the real doer.

Part of the show is our human nature with its capacities of memory and thinking which, if one takes the load of the 'past' and the 'future' upon oneself, makes the journey hard and treacherous. For the 'past' and the 'future' appear terribly big, and it is very difficult to walk along the path if one carries this load. 'If such and such actions were taken', we think, 'then a particular result could be achieved'. 'If I hadn't acted the way I did, I could have saved myself from these effects'. One should always keep oneself lighthearted and free of that burden.

In fact, the load is on the mind (*Buddhi*) itself, because the physical body has nothing to do with it; but because the mind governs the physical body, the physical body also suffers.

One of the best examples is the shadow play of puppets. There is something holding the strings and moving them, but they appear to be moving themselves and to be the real doers.

The whole creation is very much like a puppet show with the strings being held by somebody else.

In another simile, there is the example of the cinema show, where the film is being shown on the screen and people keep looking at these moving pictures. On the screen you see mountains, buildings, seas and fights, love scenes and religious scenes. All types of scenes are being enacted on this screen. Some people watching are like the puppets, and they get animated by the scenes.

One should be able to see the things which are happening in the world – but only as a silent observer. See all the pleasures on the screen, but don't be involved and move off course.

All the exciting things which are shown on the screen do not colour the screen itself, the screen is pure white. It has no colour of its own, it just reflects the colours which are thrown on it.

So we should become like a screen where all the activity takes place, is allowed to take place, but we should become pure white and not be stained by any of the colours of the world. It is not one's business to have any ambition or desire to initiate a new line of action. The flow of the *Gunas* (*Sattva, Rajas* and *Tamas*) should be experienced dispassionately.

You mentioned the dream state. There are five states: the *Samadhi* state, the awakened state, the dreaming state, and then deep sleep, and the fifth one is the unconscious state. All these five states are the mysterious creative art of the Absolute. Each of these states is part of the creation manifested for the pleasure of the Self, and in fact each state is useful for one or the other purpose. There is nothing to choose between one or another. One doesn't have to choose anything, but stand at the middle and see both sides. Just the passing life – the play of 'past' and 'future'. Each state is part of the Absolute, and one does not have to select one of these situations. One has to become the impartial and silent observer of whatever happens, may it be *Samadhi*, awake, dream or sleep. If that is achieved, it is beyond all these states of the world we live in, and in effect everything is *Sat-Chit-Ananda* – the Absolute. Even the most ordinary work, such as digging, then gives bliss (*Ananda*).

With the idea of enjoying the whole creation with this impartial attitude, one might ask where is the sense of being good? What is good and bad? The question never gets resolved. In fact, there is neither good nor bad, it is simply our nomenclature. It is our *preference* for one or the other which makes one good and the other bad, our impertinence which makes one good and the other bad.

If one could keep to this state of silent, impartial observer, one would see that none of these things exist. One stays in the present, and one acts as the occasion demands and the whole thing passes. Wise men once discussed this question of deriving *Ananda* out of all the multifarious aspects of the world, and the discussion led to the conclusion that one should not entangle oneself with either side (physical or subtle), but should simply observe; because the Absolute is in everything and this creation is a most efficient mechanical organism which is functioning by the wish of the Absolute, so one should always see the Absolute behind all these passing phases.

> One of the listeners at this discussion went away and on the road saw an elephant coming along. He remembered that the Absolute was in everything, so he thought, 'the Absolute is in the elephant, so surely it won't harm me.' The *mahout* on the elephant's back kept shouting to him to get out of the way, but the man on the road took no notice, and the elephant took him up and threw him to

one side. He went back to the wise man to say he had been misinformed – he thought the elephant was the Absolute, and he was the Absolute and the Absolute would not harm the Absolute in any way – but it did.

Then he was told, 'You did not realise that the *mahout* was also the Absolute. Because you did not obey the Absolute when he shouted to you, you were punished. You, in fact, selected one of the two. Do not select, do not show prejudice, do not make impertinent preferences. Then everything will be clear and you will find your way easily without any hindrance!'

Once Swami Rama Tirtha, who was from the Punjab, saw a black adder in his path; it was a puff adder with his hood open. He just smiled and laughed and said, 'Oh my God, you have come before me in such a frightening shape – but, forgive me, I don't like your shape this time, so please go away!' And the puff adder went away.

This shows how to behave as an unprejudiced and silent observer who has no duality (no mental division into 'good' and 'evil').

Question from RA
His Holiness has told us that the Mantra, the meditator and the object of meditation (the Universal Self) should all become one. I should like further guidance on this. With me at times the meditation stops, my personal identity ceases to exist and there is only Universal Being. Is this what His Holiness refers to?

HH: In meditation the meditator, the act of meditation and the Mantra should all become one, should be united in one. This state of unity can only be recognised by one effect during the meditation – that there is no knowledge of any sort derived from such a deep meditation. If there is still even a feeling of the Universal Being, that would mean that the ultimate stage has not yet been reached because some knowledge remains. However great and universal and refined these feelings may be, the meditation is not complete. The unity is very much like the great ocean undisturbed by waves and where the bottom of the ocean and the surface are all one.

One might enquire what is the usefulness of this stillness where there is no knowledge, and what do we do after we have meditated?

In the unified state where there is no meditator and no act of meditation, one is directly connected with the creative force of the Absolute. It is a resting point for the *Atman*, and for the *Atman* alone, to come in direct contact, not impeded, particularly by the subtle body which is the instrument of knowledge. So one would see that in the unified state there is no knowledge, not even of the Universal Being. The subtle body is what recalls all these experiences, but the unified state is the real state of the *Atman*, and one should reach that. Then, when one comes out of meditation, one would see that during all the activities of the world one does not identify oneself with mind, hand, foot, etc. One remains the *Atman* and gets all these servants to work for the *Atman*.

Take the labourer who works in the field under a supervisor. The supervisor does not work. If the supervisor works there is no supervision and chaos would follow.

So in order to become the real supervisor one should meditate and become the master of all the labourers, *Manas*, *Buddhi* and

Chitta. These are the labourers, and we must become still to get the most out of these labourers in our organism.

His Holiness concluded by saying that during the discourses we must keep a constant vigil and probe the questions and the answers and pursue anything that is not clear.

ALLAHABAD 1972
Second Audience
Wednesday 4 October

Question from FCR

About the ladder of Self-realisation. Twelve years ago when, after a year of meditation, we came to Rishikesh, some of us were speaking only of the seventh step. Later, at Lucknow and here, I kept asking about the fourth and fifth steps. Now I want to ask about the first steps. We get many good impulses and we make plenty of good resolutions, but we don't carry them through. I want the energy and the will power to carry through that resolution from which one never goes back – that the Universal Self should be all in all during each day as it is when one first wakes from deep and dreamless sleep.

HH: You asked about the good impulses and all the good resolutions which come in one's everyday life and then are not usually carried through. One has to differentiate between two types of good resolutions and good impulses. One is born of the mind (*Manas*) and is the effect of time and place, of certain situations or certain influences which come from outside. We seem to be *in* those situations, so we resolve to do certain things. The other is born of understanding (*Buddhi*), which comprehends that in such and such a situation we have this much energy or capacity; and so, with this capacity, we resolve to take up an activity or any one of the good resolutions, and then we carry it through. We do not just drop it because times have changed, the atmosphere is gone or our energy is dissipated. So one has to decide by one's own reason as to whether the resolutions to be taken are worthwhile, whether they can be carried through; and then, once having decided, we should keep to these resolutions.

Question from FCR
According to His Holiness's answer yesterday it is the *Param-Atman* doing and we are just trying to prevent something coming in between the Will of the *Param-Atman* and the role we have to play?

HH: In a telephone exchange there are thousands and thousands of lines available, and people in different places have their telephones installed; but the lines are available only for the asking. You have to ask for the number to get connected.

Of the same sort is this Manifested Nature (*Prakriti*), which is three-fold: *Sattvic, Rajasic* and *Tamasic*. One only has to ask for any of these *Sattvic, Rajasic* and *Tamasic* influences to be given to one and they would be available. The individual is also composed of these three facets of the *Prakriti* and so is the whole universe, for the *Param-Atman* has manifested this creation through these three *Gunas*. So the process works automatically. If one asks from the heart for anything, it should be available; and one can carry on according to one's good resolution – provided one really continues to want it.

One will sometimes see that situations are not favourable for one's good resolutions or good impulses, and they will fail – not because one doesn't want to carry them through, but because present circumstances do not allow them to be carried through, and one is handicapped by a situation which is not under one's control.

The Absolute, who governs everything, knows properly what is most necessary for certain situations, so even if resolutions are not being carried through, one should accept the situation as part of the Grace of the Absolute, even if it is in opposition to one's resolution. In due course things will change and go the way you want. To have good resolutions is not a part of worldly desire, it is of the Divine Nature. One must wait until the proper turn of *Prakriti* makes circumstances available for the individual to carry through his resolutions.

Comment from FCR

This answer relates to my own desire to cease from teaching others, but I remember a higher example when His Holiness had once said that he did not want to be in public life for more than twelve years, but circumstances forced this upon him.

Question from RA

His Holiness says we should ask from the heart, how do we do this?

HH: There is a simple solution to the problem of knowing whether the resolution comes from the heart – a resolution coming from the heart stays with the heart. Any resolution which is lost in time is not from the heart.

Question from RA

But in the example of the telephone exchange, His Holiness said you only have to ask and the line will be made available to you, provided you ask from the heart. This is not quite the same as resolution, is it? We form questions in the mind, but how do we communicate in this way from the heart?

HH: The good resolutions from the heart spring from within, and that which springs from within keeps on reminding one again and again. The other type of resolution, which flashes into the mind, is the result of certain situations and associations.

When these associations and situations are gone, then those resolutions are also lost in time. So one has to see if some idea or resolution is reminding one again and again in spite of all difficulties and opposing situations; then this is proved to be coming from the heart and must be kept going, and, in fact, you will be forced to keep this going simply because it comes from the heart.

As an example: If you have to go to a far distant city in a car, when you come to a small town you have to slow down the speed of the car because of the traffic conditions in the town. In the heart of the city you have to go slower still, and you may even have to stop for some time and start again. When the road is clear, you can go faster to reach your destination.

In the same way, when resolutions come from the heart, situations may delay their fulfilment, but the speed can be increased again when better circumstances allow it. However, if it comes from the mind, and is checked, you will not remember it and it will be lost.

Question from RA
His Holiness mentioned yesterday the spiritual influences which are available here. Is there anything we can do to make them available in equal strength in London?

HH: Yes, of course, this is quite possible, but it can only be done in the normal way:

If we want to plant a tree and get fruit, we always start from the seed or a sapling, and we look after it to allow it to grow and provide all necessary conditions without any disturbance, and in course of time it takes root, grows, and eventually you can enjoy the fruit. So everything is available later on.

It is just like an infectious disease which spreads because people come into contact. So it is with spiritual influences – they also spread only after people come in contact with you; so the best thing one can do is to have more contact where one lives, and slowly, when the influences which you have collected from here are passed on to other people, they will keep on multiplying and increasing. In this way it would be possible for your own place to become spiritually impregnated with such influences, and then everybody can make use of them. It is much like an electric current and this story illustrates it.

> There was once a trader who was very afraid of thieves getting into his shop to steal his cash at night. He therefore had his safe connected to the electric current to make it alive, and each night he would switch on, and disconnect it next morning.
> One night four thieves got through the back door and one of them touched the safe and could not move. Another said, 'Why are you not moving?' and went to pull him away, but he also became stuck to the first. The third tried to pull away the first two and also became stuck, and likewise the fourth. So all were stuck and died because of the electric current. In the morning the trader came to open the shop and saw this, and informed the police and explained that, since he was afraid of thieves, he had connected his safe to the electric current.

This story is only to illustrate that good influences can also be given to people, but it has to be done in a systematic way by constant contact with the people. In India the good influences which are available are the product of thousands of years of this devotional work which has kept going in India all this time.

For thousands of years in India this tradition of the spiritual life had taken root, and quite a number of people used to devote their full life to the search of the spiritual mystery in two ways. One way was to look into the spiritual life and attain spirituality through the medium of *action*. The other was to renounce the world – not by any action – but work for liberation by complete *detachment*. Now, whatever differences there were between these two groups, they needed to support each other, and the whole fabric of society was interwoven with these two systems. So a young man would have to go through one of these two systems in his student life, and before he came out into the householder's life he would have received influences and training and knowledge so that he could live a good moral life in the world.

But now, even in India, this oral influence of the spiritual realm is lost to a great extent. It is now available only in a few centres where the Tradition remains alive. The average Indian is now so intent on the search for material gain that he is not at all interested in the spiritual way of life. Yet after some time, when more material gain has been achieved, it will again be found that the spiritual side is lacking and that material gain alone does not bring real happiness. The tide will turn again and only then will this Tradition, which is enshrined in some places, spread again.

This modern time is such that the material gain is the foremost thing in the mind of the people everywhere, but again, in India, there are still certain people engaged in keeping this Tradition alive and making these influences available only to those who want them. When the proper time comes, then these influences will increase in India. In the same way, if you collect influences from here and have more contact with people in your own country, then these influences can be spread.

Question from FCR
At my lectures in New York people asked me why I had to go to India – so far away! I told them it was not geographical, but accomplishment in Self-realisation. I knew what I wanted, and if I could have found it nearer home it would have been more convenient. I went on to mention His Holiness's example of the lame man and the blind man. Would His Holiness have suggested something better?

HH: The simile of the lame man and the blind man is quite all right. According to Indian tradition this story is related to the Natural Law and the man-made law.

Man-made law does not have far sight, and the Natural Law does not have the capacity to command because it simply moves on naturally; whereas the man-made law commands, demands and makes people follow it, but does not have far sight of any sort. So, although the blind man can walk and work, he cannot see far ahead, whereas the Natural Law, which has the far sight, does not have the legs, so it cannot move by itself.

In the worldly life the combination of these two is necessary, so that the movement towards the achievement of Self-realisation and liberation is possible – only by the union of the lame and blind. It works by this union because the regulations become a little more gentle and people can be moved by the gentle touch of Natural Law, rather than being coerced by man-made regulations to do certain things by force. The achievements are bigger with the man-made laws, but they do not last long.

Question from MA
One looks forward so much to coming here and as I said yesterday one feels one has been spiritually lazy, and the more pleasant the life has been the bigger the debt one feels, but I see from His Holiness's answer yesterday this is just an excuse. But I would like to ask the difference between laziness and passivity during meditation, because one feels the need for greater passivity to get to the depth but also one can find that one is lazy and just indulging in the pleasant dreams.

HH: The situation described implies that, if one finds oneself lazy on the way, then there is some sort of regret for being lazy, or some sort of despondency for having done something wrong. This is the main cause of developing despondency and reverting back to the inferior influences. Even if the situations are in opposition and you are not able to carry on whatever you think you should have done, don't regret – just look ahead and see if they can be done now.

In the life of individuals they have to work according to a certain plan, and it is not necessary for the plan to be achieved in one day. In one day they have to take food, clean their body, arrange their room and do all sorts of other works, and earn their livelihood. Doing all these things every day, they carry out this plan day after day, every morning. In the spiritual life also, if a good resolution has been taken, such as mentioned by MA about the debt, this debt will be completed only if one keeps on doing it every day; and if some day or other period of time was passed in lazy activities, one should not regret, but rather look happily ahead to doing it again.

Suppose someone has a good impulse in the last stages of their life when there is neither the energy nor the time to fulfil this resolution. Should one regret in such a situation? No, it is not necessary. Even if the body were to fall, he would certainly come back in a more favourable situation to take up the resolution from the past life.

In the *Bhagavad Gita* also it has been said that if a Yogi dies before full Realization, he is born in a very favoured set-up to complete the work. This is quite obvious for one sees every day that in the search for Divine life or liberation there are both elderly and young seekers of spiritual Truth. Sometimes young boys or girls also seem to be much interested and involved in this work. This is only because in their previous or present life a good impulse has set them working. Let the work proceed and progress as it naturally does and, if any shortcoming is seen, just see it and forget it and don't regret it. But do make the best use of the next moment which comes before you with full hope and possibility to support your resolution.

Question from DC
Dr DC has been asked to give lectures to young doctors about 'understanding human behaviour' and asks what His Holiness would consider important in talking to them about this subject.

HH: The study of human behaviour is best done by those who have studied the spiritual life. The spiritual life teaches one to look at oneself, so those who have looked at themselves would be able to appreciate far more quickly the behaviour of other people.

When we are buying something we only look at a sample, and then we are satisfied that the material delivered to the house would be exactly the same as the sample.

So one does not have to study individuals for years and years. Twenty-four hours are enough to indicate the type of person he is, and in twenty-four hours he will show different examples of *Rajas, Tamas.* He will show everything, and one can watch and find out where this individual is trying to proceed, at what level he is, what his ambitions are, and what the future is for him. One can study individuals only if one studies oneself.

Take the example of a doctor who has learnt the art of medicine. A patient comes before him who may be suffering from many diseases simultaneously. An efficient doctor immediately finds out which is the main disease and which are the subsidiary ones which follow in its wake. He treats the main disease first, and then looks after the other ones.

In human behaviour there are certain main facets one has to look for. Having seen these, all the secondary things which come after can be studied. The study of human behaviour can only be done by those who study themselves.

75

ALLAHABAD 1972
Third Audience, Thursday 5 October

Question from JR

It seems to me that His Holiness is trying to get us to understand that, by dwelling on our shortcomings and deficiencies, we are preventing the power of *Param-Atman* from reaching us.

HH: Your observation is right – all activities which are initiated by an individual are aimed at some sort of gain (gain not in the bad sense but personal advancement) and whenever one takes to any thinking about one's deeds then one gets involved with that deed, and creates a sort of identity between something that happened previously with the person who ponders about it. Since a mistake has been made, you are tying yourself to the mistake. All mistakes are taking away precious energy which could equally be used for better actions. So if you keep thinking about your mistakes or shortcomings in the past, then you are wasting energy.

If you can get rid of that activity, then it would be possible for you to *engage your attention on the next moment*, a process which promises to bring you extra energy by merging with the Absolute or *Param-Atman*, or any action related to the *Param-Atman*.

Sunday 8 October

Question from RA

Last Wednesday the Guru referred to the search for spirituality through the medium of action and the medium of renunciation. Could he say more about the medium of action?

HH: As I said before, there are two different ways of approaching the liberation of mankind from human form. One is through activity towards liberation, and the other is by renunciation – complete renunciation of the worldly life, and withdrawing oneself into such corners where one is not obliged to attend to any activity of the world. Of course he will attend to activity related to liberation but not related to the world. There are certain examples of this: Rama, Vasishtha and Janaka.

Note: Rama was the incarnation of God who was the hero of the great Hindu epic, the Ramayana. *King Janaka you have heard of through the stories His Holiness tells about him. Vashishta we know little about, but the following words of Shri Ramakrishna refer to him:*

'He who has knowledge has ignorance also. "How amazing", said Lakshman to Rama, "even a sage like Vashishta was stricken with grief because of the death of his sons!" "My brother", replied Rama, "he who has knowledge has ignorance also. Therefore go beyond both knowledge and ignorance."'

His Holiness said, in 1967, 'The teacher also never claims anything for himself, because he knows that he is also just one of the links in the chain of disciple-teacher relationship in this Tradition, which started from the first teacher called Narayana (a name of the god Vishnu) and passed through Brahma, Vasishtha, Sri Shankara, and so on, up to the present time.'

HH: These three examples are exponents of this philosophy of liberation through activity. They were householders who were very famous men. One of the main facets of worldly anxiety is the fear and pressure attached to birth and death. By themselves they have nothing to do with any sort of bondage –

it is only when one takes them very seriously and treats them as real, then the bondage starts and the trouble appears. A man of activity would learn to discern what the reality behind the appearance is and, although he would act in the appearance, he would always hold on to the reality and thus avoid the conflict of pleasure and displeasure which seems to appear through birth and death.

For example, one knows, and everyone knows, that one is a human being, and this human being, neither in his awake state nor in his dream state, or sleep or any other state, would ever think that he was not a man – he would never consider himself a beast of any sort. In the same way, if one knew precisely and decisively that one is the *Atman* or the Absolute, then there is no reason to by-pass any worldly activities, one can sail through them by virtue of reason, *discernment*[†], and act as the situation demands and hold no *Sanskar*[‡] for it.

It is the birthright of human beings to walk on the earth but it is not necessary that they must also swim in the water, but they can *learn* to swim, and if they have learnt to swim they can walk or swim, whatever the circumstances may be. They will be able to do their job or cross the land or the river whenever it is necessary. It is in exactly the same way that the human being can learn to swim through the world into the liberated land and act whenever the action is needed from him. This is the householder's way.

FCR handed the following to interpreter Dixit for translation and submission to His Holiness:

[†] dis + cerno = I sift (giving rise to insight).
[‡] Sanskaras, qualities and effects passed on from life to life

Mathematics and physics in the West have become so complicated that they bear little relation to the practical life of the householder. But recently we have had one or two university professors in those subjects doing the meditation with much benefit. It would be useful if we could prove to them that ancient wisdom (for example, about the laws of three and seven) could solve their problems more simply. You will, of course, know the following story with which we could perhaps begin, if our version is accurate:

There lived long ago, in the country of King Dharmasana, an old Brahmin who had three sons, and who possessed nothing in the world but 19 cows. Before he died he called his sons and said, 'My Sons, I am in the mouth of death, so listen attentively. All I have to give you are these 19 cows; divide them among you in this way: let the eldest take half of them, the middle son a quarter, and the youngest a fifth share of them. But should there be any remainder left over, you must all three of you eat it, if not, all the cows are to be given to the king and my curse will rest upon you.' And saying this the old Brahmin died.

When, after performing the rites of burial, they came together to divide the property, the eldest brother said, 'Half of these cows, that is, nine cows and a half are mine.' The next brother said, 'One quarter, that is, four cows and three-fourths of a cow are mine.' And the youngest said, 'The remaining fifth, that is, three cows and four-fifths of a cow are mine.'

The eldest then remarked, 'But the sum of all these added together amounts only to eighteen cows and a fraction of a cow. But how is it possible for Brahmins to eat the flesh of a cow, or how are we to take various pieces of a cow and leave it still alive? But unless we share in due measure, all the cows must go to the king and our father's curse will fall on us. Why did our father place us in so terrible a dilemma?'

After debating day and night, they at last put their problem to a holy man. After a moment's thought he replied, 'Let the brothers borrow another cow. Then of the 20 cows, let the eldest take half, or ten cows; the next a quarter, or five cows; and the youngest a fifth, or four cows. Then let them return the borrowed cow. Thus the 19 cows will be divided according to the father's instructions, with no remainder. Each brother will receive more than by their own division, and finally the king will be pleased. For he is a just king, and what would displease him more than that, anywhere in his kingdom, Brahmins should kill and eat cows, let alone chop them up, and, at the same time, disregard their father's dying instructions?'

Note by FCR: I used to think only that this story was a key to the Laws of Nature, for Nature always prefers whole numbers to fractions. But lately I perceive another meaning also, that whenever we put any problem, however complex, to the Param-Atman or to His representative, the fully Realised man, the answer comes back in so new and simple a form that one gasps, 'Why couldn't I have thought of that?'

Reply from His Holiness
The mathematicians and the physicists should understand that in the Laws of Nature there are no 'oddities' anywhere. There is, on the other hand, an 'evenness' throughout. That is why they are so amenable to reason, and ultimately they all fit into one another

so simply and beautifully. Ancient wisdom does help to solve problems easily. It is all contained in ancient 'Granthas' (books). But by simply reading them nobody can solve the problems as the 'Granthas' contain 'Granthis' (knots) which can only be opened by experienced *Gurus*.

For example, if arsenic is prescribed for the treatment of a particular disease, it takes a medical man to say in what form and in what dosage the arsenic is to be given.

These 'Granthis' or knots are sometimes introduced purposefully.

> A rich man built a temple. On the Vijay Dashma day and at four o'clock in the evening, he buried four pots full of gold coins just where the shadow of the temple's pinnacle fell on the ground. He left a note in his will for his sons stating that he had buried four pots full of gold coins at four o'clock on the Vijay Dashma day at the pinnacle of the temple, and that they may take it out if and when they ran into financial difficulties.
>
> Eventually the sons did run into financial difficulties. They broke the pinnacle and found nothing. Then they dug out the whole temple in search of the pots, still getting nothing. As they were in trouble for want of money, they talked to everyone about it. One day a Mahatma passed that way and he also heard their problem. After inspecting the site carefully, he asked them to rebuild the temple just as it was. This was easily done as all the materials of the old temple were lying there. Then he asked them to call him again on the day of the festival of Vijaya-dashami [start of the harvest season] and they did so.

He saw where the shadow of the temple's pinnacle fell at four o'clock on that day, and asked the sons to dig there. The pots were found after digging down only a few feet.

Regarding the story of the Brahmin and his sons, it has a psychological meaning also. The five organs of action, plus the five organs of sense, plus the five '*pranas*', together with *Manas*, *Buddhi*, *Chitta* and *Ahankara* make nineteen, and they constitute the body of the sons which the Brahmin left. These were the nineteen cows. The twentieth cow, which was borrowed and which facilitates the division, was *Wisdom* and did not form part of the body. Naturally it was left out as it only facilitated the division and it did not actually enter it.

Further comment by FCR

This 'illuminating' answer confirms the idea of 'wisdom' as a *catalyst*, which makes a chemical reaction possible, but it is not used up itself in the process – the borrowed cow! It also illustrates the method of the Calculus which uses 'infinitesimals' in the process of differentiation and then, by integration, removes them and reinserts the 'constant'.

ALLAHABAD 1972
Last Audience
Friday 13 October

Question from FCR
First, we wish to thank you for the wonderful feast you spread before us yesterday with, I believe, 24 different dishes. We were even able to enjoy a few second helpings to make up for the absence of Mr Allan!

But now I ask your Holiness for what you wish to say, and ask for your instructions.

HH: In the Indian Tradition the *Vedas* are the source of all types of knowledge that are available in India, and the *Vedas* contain support for all aspects of approach to the Absolute. In fact, according to one's own inclinations and preferences one can find support in the *Vedas* to establish the validity of the Absolute, and the purity of the ways and means adopted to reach the Absolute are all available. Just as human beings have different tastes and preferences in food – some liking sweet, some savoury, some salty, some bitter – and they always look for and improve upon these tastes, by this they quench their thirst and hunger and enjoy it. None of these tastes is better or worse than others, it is a question of the inclination which creates and opens up a way of realising the Absolute.

As has been told often before, there are primarily three Ways: the Way of *Karma* (Action), the Way of *Jnana* (Knowledge), and the Way of *Bhakti* (Devotion).

So there are people who can appreciate and devote their time and energy to the intellectual pursuit of the Absolute, and it is this one aspect of the Absolute which they prefer and like to work with and become One with that aspect, and for which they are equipped so that it suits them. They cannot go any other Way. Similarly, there are people who cannot appreciate the intellect and they like to work on the emotions, and through the emotional pursuit they seek to become One with that aspect, so if there are intellectual discussions, they usually shy off and prefer only those things related to emotional work. Also there are those who cannot go either through the intellect or by devotion, and who prefer to do something practical. So there are three Ways to approach the Absolute, and none of them is better or worse than the others.

The *Vedas* are supposed to be the most authoritative collection of the Scriptures. Everything has to be referred to the *Vedas*. Only if it is supported by the *Vedas* can a System be honoured in India. So everybody tries to look to the *Vedas* for threads of support. In the *Vedas*, and particularly the *Upanishads*, it says in one place that without knowledge it is not possible for one to attain liberation. All those people who are inclined to the intellectual way have always quoted this part of the *Vedic* text to show that nobody, whoever he may be, who has not learnt about the Absolute and learnt the knowledge thoroughly, can liberate his soul from the duality of birth and death.

Similarly, there are quotations given by devotional people, taken from the *Vedas*, to show that without devotion no liberation is possible, and they say, 'After all, knowledge is only a dry thing, and what use is knowledge to anyone. It is only through devotion one should approach the Absolute – forget all knowledge and forget all activity!'.

But all the adherents of activity can also quote certain things from the *Vedas* to show that, unless you put the teaching into practice by performing right action, nothing will happen; for Self-realisation, arduous physical disciplines are required, so all your knowledge and devotions are of no use unless you express them in performing your day-to-day obligations.[†]

Common man, hearing quotations from all these three sources, usually gets perplexed, for he is neither fully capable of all activity, nor of all knowledge, nor can he fully devote himself to the Absolute because he has to live his householder's life. There alone is the need for enquiry for anyone who, after hearing different views and being perplexed, should get everything clear for his own sake.

Here is an example :

> Once in a village an elephant arrived and the news went around so everyone wanted to see the elephant. Unfortunately most of the inhabitants were blind, and yet they had the desire to experience the elephant, so

---

[†]His Holiness had previously explained that the *Bhagavad Gita*, which is the cream of all the *Vedas*, is based on these three: the first six chapters being devoted to the Yoga of Action (*Karma*), the next six to the Yoga of Devotion (*Bhakti*), and the last six to the Yoga of Knowledge (*Jnana*).

they were led to it. The *mahout* (man in charge of the elephant) let them explore the elephant by touching it, and of course each one touched a different part. Having made their investigations they assembled together and wanted to verify that they had experienced the real thing. The one who felt the foot said an elephant was a pillar, the one who had felt the tail said the elephant was like a stick, and so it went on with the ears, trunk, tusks, fat tummy, etc., each describing it according to the type of previous experience to which they could relate it. Then they started refuting each other – 'Yours was not the proper elephant, yours was an illusion, mine is the only real one', etc.

Later, the *mahout* told them, 'You cannot actually have a complete vision of the elephant. All you can really do is put together all these different personal experiences of 'elephant', and from them a novel creature can be imagined which is known as 'elephant'. But it is the sum of all these parts and *something more*, which represents the unity of the creature known as elephant.'

In the same way, because of the different quotations from the Scriptures, it is possible and it is usual for some sort of conflict or doubt to arise in the minds of people. They must make an effort to get it clarified because there are people like this *mahout* in our spiritual life who are able to dispel their doubts.

Question from FCR
May we speak of one or two more subjects close to our hearts? To us four and many of our friends there is no longer any difference in our soul (*Antahkarana*) between *Param-Atman*, the present Shankaracharya, and the great men of his Tradition or

our Christian Tradition. They are all one and the same. If we call constantly on *Param-Atman* for help in any problem, something of all that you have said comes to our help. For instance, your recent answer to Mr. Rabeneck: 'A feeling of sameness possesses our heart with eyes open or shut. The mind sheds its burdens and becomes filled with joy instead.'

HH: Your observation is very good, and since it happens like that, it is commendable. The Tradition of the Shankaracharya was started from Narayana; as you know, that means the Absolute Himself; and then was followed by others like Vyasa, Gandapadacharya and then the original Shankara, and after him hundreds of Shankaracharyas right down to the one you are facing. It is quite possible that even the Shankaracharyas, according to their own being, may have had certain preferences and would have invoked these Vedic Scriptures to support their particular way, but in fact they all lead to the same ultimate end. There is no difference of ideology underlying them, in support of man's search for liberation. There may be little preferences which can be different. There was a man called Madhusudan Saraswati. He was a Shankarite. He belonged to the Shankaracharya system and was one of the greatest intellectual giants of the latter Middle Ages of India, but he had a preference for Devotion, so all his books have an under-lying support for Devotion in preference to the Way of Knowledge. Although he, himself, was a man of knowledge, he supported the Devotional Way.

In the same way, all that has been propounded here through His Holiness, is in fact not his, but belongs to the Tradition, so all this traditional work and the Knowledge which goes through Dr Roles or Mr Allan or others in their own way, is related to the same Tradition. It is not the individuals who speak, but the Tradition speaks through these individuals.

Question from FCR
Lately, in a letter, His Holiness reminded us that the world, either as we see it in dreams or in the waking state, has three stages, creation, maintenance and destruction. In my understanding, it is the middle one which we don't know the real meaning of, or what it is about. Somehow, in my heart, the idea of Lord Vishnu is connected with this. If I read anything about Vishnu or his incarnations, it refreshes and cheers me. Such as the story of Ajamila in the *Bhagavatam*.

HH: These three steps or situations which you describe, creation, maintenance and destruction, these are the aspects of the three *Gunas: Sattva, Rajas* and *Tamas*. Vishnu belongs to the state of *Sattva*, Brahma to the *Rajas* and Rudra or Shiva to the *Tamas*. In *Rajas* there is no fixed position or state. *Rajas* is not stable, it is not a materialisation of anything, it is activity when things are about to take shape. The state comes either in the *Sattvic* region or in the *Tamasic* region, and it is only because of this that Brahma in India has never been worshipped and is never favoured for any worship anywhere in India – except only in the Yagya (when a sacrifice has to be performed). Since Brahma is the Creator, he is the first ancestor, he is the great-great-grandfather of all human beings, so at most he is offered a seat of honour at the sacrifice and given oblations so as to please him. Otherwise he is never given any preference or devotion. Whenever you take to activity, there are only two positions. Either you will get tired and exhausted and go to sleep (*Tamas*), rest there and come out later on; or, after putting yourself into active form and having achieved the end of the activity and everything materialises in success, then, in return, you get the bliss or enjoyment (*Sattva*) of having done the job well and successfully. This enjoyment immediately gives light, makes you light, and you feel very fresh even after strenuous work.

Now yesterday, at your feast here, all the people who were engaged in preparation of the food, were very eager to see how their labour fared. When they saw the smiling faces of those for whom the food was made, and they saw the appreciation of the food, they were delighted – a lot more than any of you who enjoyed the food. In return this created far more bliss, and all their exertion was finished and they enjoyed the occasion far more than you could have done. This is how it works. So Vishnu is related to this sustaining of this universe, and he sustains only by giving something – just as the food was prepared for you like a sacrifice in honour of the guests – and with love Vishnu maintains the whole creation. Vishnu is one of the deities most honoured in Indian tradition because of the protection and sustenance he offers through love.

Question from FCR

I particularly like the story of Ajamila because here is a man who started well but led a sinful life, and when faced with death he was very frightened, but he pronounced the name of Narayana (the name of his favourite son) so the attendants of Vishnu came and sent away the attendants of death, and I myself had a similar experience!

HH: In Indian history, as put in the *Bhagavatam*, the role of the Holy men – the Mahatmas – is very important. Mahatmas have a life of their own, but they appear in common life as well, and when they appear in common life they always come with advice – some sort of tactful advice – so that without disturbing the life of the common man or his frame of mind, they put in something which is of direct use to the individual, even though he does not realise the importance of the advice given to him. The story of Ajamila is an example of this tactful, practical advice:

He was an ordinary man engaged in his worldly life and not of any saintly disposition. Once a Mahatma happened to come by his town and to eat at his house and wanted, in return, to give him some tactful advice. So the Mahatma asked him, 'what is it that attracts you most? Is there anything to which you are, above all, attached?'

Ajamila said, 'I am most attached to my youngest son.' So the Mahatma asked him to give the youngest son the name of Narayana. Whenever, therefore, he had to call this boy, he should call him by that name, and so he did.

There wasn't anything more that Ajamila was asked to do. He wasn't prescribed any discipline or *satsang* or other things, except this advice. So at the time of his death, as usual, without knowing, he called Narayana his little son and because of this name the messengers of Narayana (Vishnu) appeared and liberated him.

In the course of devotional work which people do, for instance, in India there are temples with carved stone statues of gods before which people worship, bow down and pray. In fact, it is not the stone sculpture which is being worshipped, it is the *idea* of the God which has been superimposed on this stone statue, and it is because of the devotion to the particular idea of God that they get attuned to that God. But as far as the names are concerned, the

Mantras, they are very potent even though there is no form attached to the Mantra. In fact, the name Narayana stood for a Mantra which, without being initiated, he used to recite in calling his son. Just as in meditation we are given certain words, the word has no form other than the vocal sound. It is not attached to any particular deity, or any particular meaning, it is only a sound, but it is a creative sound.

All sounds are creative, so when a Mantra is given, this creative sound becomes the vehicle of transformation in the individual. Thus, because Ajamila used to pronounce the name Narayana, which is very like a Mantra, the forces involved in the sound were made use of for his Self-development. Just as with fire, if you touch it, whether knowingly or unknowingly, then it is bound to burn you, to hurt you. In exactly the same way, a Mantra like Ram and Narayana, whether you know anything about it or not, if you utter it, it will come to the rescue and do the job of liberation or whatever it can.

FCR: We wish His Holiness success in his visit to the Himalayas (of which we read in today's newspaper) and we want to thank him very much for all his patience with us at this time, and may we continue to write – not expecting answers!

His Holiness nods and offers his blessings for the development of all those souls scattered all over the world under your leadership. May they prosper.

During these audiences, at HH's order, one of the Sannyasins of the Ashram, Dandi Swami, who spoke excellent English, answered questions and told a number of stories.

Question from RA to Dandi Swami
You told us that the past and future is already printed on the cinema reel. Are the meetings that I have had with His Holiness and now with you, and whatever may follow from these meetings, also already recorded on the reel of my life, or is it possible that such an occurrence as these meetings may change my part in the drama?

Dandi Swami: However much I may tell you that everything is predestined, or already recorded on the reel, you won't admit it because ego is there. Therefore, in spite of realising that everything is predestined, everything is being directed by God Himself, your ego won't admit it, and will go on as if it is the doer. A story illustrates this.

On a mast of a ship a bird was sitting quietly when the ship left the port and was going out to sea. The bird was confident that it could fly the distance back and reach its own place. After a long time with the ship far out to sea, it was evening, and the bird was thinking that its children would be crying for it at home, and it made an attempt to fly home across the ocean. But it could not find the shore, so thought it must have mistaken the direction and returned to the mast for a rest. When it was rested it set off again in another direction, but the same thing happened – it could not find the shore because the distance was too great. It was not within the power of the bird to reach the shore. It went to the south, to the north, to the east and west, but in the end it realised there was nothing it could do, so it returned to the mast and once more sat quietly.

Now it was confident again, but in another way, not that 'I can do', but 'I must go where the mast of the ship is taking me'.

So long as you are in the individual ego and not on the cosmic plane, you will be thinking that you can do it yourself.

Now, when I am speaking, it is only what His Holiness intends me to say. His Holiness transmits – I speak. Yesterday you said that I was speaking too fast, but the ideas which His Holiness was transmitting were so full that I was trying to transmit all of them to you.

I give the example of Vivekananda who went to New York and was told that he would only have five minutes to address an audience. He stood up intending to speak himself, and found he was dumb. But he remembered his Guru, Ramakrishna, who was dead, and suddenly the words flowed in such a way that the audience was fascinated and he was allowed to go on much longer than five minutes.

Although his Guru was dead, Cosmic Mind could make this connection. Distance and place are not a bar, nor time.

So if you put your questions direct to His Holiness he might have used different words, and answered in a very short way, but the essence would be the same. So don't think, 'I have spent all this money, and come all this way, to hear His Holiness, and this old fellow is doing all the talking.'

Question from FCR to Dandi Swami
His Holiness had given instructions to 'pray to *Param-Atman* in solitude with a settled mind', and I tried every way for some tine. But 'mind' never could do it. Then recently I found that something was praying. Who is it that prays?

Dandi Swami: There are two things called 'I' – the Great Self which is pure Consciousness, and the little self that identifies with the physical body and the senses. One wears temporary clothes, the other is pure, naked. The clothed one is praying to the naked one that he also may be naked. In the story of the lion cub, the lion had not *become* a sheep, he only thought he was a sheep. There was no physical change – only a different mental attitude.

Prayer is needed only so long as you don't see yourself in the ocean of Consciousness. But in both those states the *Param-Atman* remains unchanged.

His Holiness (intervening):
The limited one is praying to the infinite. You cannot have complete happiness when you are limited because there is still something left to desire. As long as the finite is not merged with the infinite, there will be desire, and so effort and prayer will be there.

A person once came and asked me, 'If God is omnipresent and omniscient, then whose ignorance is it?' The answer was, 'You are in truth omnipresent and omniscient, and ignorance is only forgetfulness.' So the ignorance belongs to the person who is asking the question.

Observation by FCR
I am beginning to understand also that the film is already made
– you cannot go to the cinema and ask them to change the reel.

Dandi Swami: But you can change the attitude of your mind.

ALLAHABAD 1973
28 January
Mela Talk

The word 'RAM' possesses special attractions and attributes. The trilling sound of 'RA' directs the mind to the vibrations of such vibrant forms of energy as those which live in the sun, the heavenly bodies and fire, etc, with which the drama of the universe began to take shape from nothing.

Then the sound 'M' with its humming note, calms everything down into something which words fail to express.

This is, however, only to say a little about its significance and subtle effects; though a close observation of things around us would reveal a whole series of its secrets one after another.

To take only a crude example: watch the sound of the huge furnaces of the Bhilai steel plant, which pours out torrents of molten iron. You constantly hear 'Rrm-m! Rrm-m! Rrrrr-m! ...' So, this sound emits when a hard substance like iron melts, purifies, goes into still better steel.

This would look like a far-fetched example to illustrate the point, and so would each and every example quoted individually. But considering the cumulative evidence as a whole, we are led to a more significant conclusion:

It is thus that Hanuman, by remembering the sacred Name, was able to bring under his will the great *Param-Atman*.

Valmiki, using it even with letters reversed by mistake, became himself like *Param-Atman*.

Panini, an author of immortal fame, says that as soon as a word is uttered, it creates the thought of the object it represents.

Thus 'RAM' lives in everything, in every heart, and takes every shape. It is, however, One and only One.

29 January
Mela Talk

As compared with the huge size of the universe we live in, this human body of ours is like a speck of dust. Compared with the unlimited Consciousness of the *Param-Atman*, our mind (*Buddhi*) is like a drop in the ocean. And the problem before us is how to tackle that great Consciousness with such limited means – a hopeless business apparently! But hope comes from the saying, 'God helps those that help themselves', which is fortunately true!

The real cause of failure is not the inadequate means, but an inadequacy of understanding and of determination. Provided we understand what is required, and provided our determination (to shed the burden we carry) is strong enough, a very little can achieve great results, because on seeing the invincibility of our determination, the heart of *Param-Atman* melts and He Himself comes to our help.

> This is illustrated by the story of the two birds whose eggs were washed away by the sea. They made up their minds to fill up the sea. They picked up drops of seawater in their tiny beaks and dropped them on the

beach, and from there they picked up some sand and dropped it in the sea. This went on for some time. Seeing them doing this, other birds also joined them till it became a curious sight to see.

Rishi Agastya happened to pass that way, and on seeing such fun going on he enquired what it was all about. The birds told him their story.

'Do you really think', asked the Rishi, 'that you could complete this work even by labouring all your life, night and day?'

'No. But we are determined to devote not only this life, but a thousand lives, or even more, to this work until it is completed. We are resolved that we are not going to put up with the injustice that the sea has perpetrated on our innocent offspring.'

The Rishi was moved by the just cause of the birds and their strong determination to recover their eggs from the sea. He used his Yogic powers to restore the birds' eggs to them.

This is a standard story, always quoted to illustrate how strong your determination should be if you are small and your task great.

All doctrines and scriptures say that *Param-Atman* can be reached by going through some established system of discipline. But we see people who have tried them all and yet achieved nothing. The reason is that, for union with the pure Consciousness of *Param-Atman*, we cannot lay down any laws as Newton did for the physical universe, and then feel sure that everything will go accordingly. The union with *Param-Atman* is achieved solely by His grace, when His heart melts on seeing the rock-like determination of the devotee.

An Aryan Samajista (a sect which, among other things, condemns idolatry) and an idol-worshipping devotee used to live side by side. Day in and day out the former pestered the latter to give up idol worship and to start praying to the all-pervading and omnipotent God. Eventually this pestering became unbearable to the devotee and he made a sincere prayer to his deity, Krishna, to deliver him from his troublesome neighbour.

Then Krishna showed himself to the Aryan Samajista in a dream, but he denounced him in the dream and told him that he recognised no Krishna at all. When he woke up, he saw a vision of Krishna before his eyes. He turned his head away from it but in whichever direction he looked he saw the same vision. This sent him out of his wits. Telling all this to the devotee, he apologised to him for his previous conduct.

The devotee wept before the deity and prayed, distraught that the Master had not shown himself to him despite all his years of devotion, and instead appeared before the other man who denounced him. Then Krishna also appeared to him in a dream and consoled him that what he did was at his own request.

There are seven successive stages like the steps of a ladder, each leading to the next, till the final stage is reached. They are:

1. The first stage is *good actions*, which lead to
2. the second stage, which is *good thoughts*.
3. Good thoughts lead to the third stage which is *decrease in bad thoughts*.
4. Decrease in bad thoughts leads to the fourth stage which is when *Sattva predominates*.

5. This 'energy of *Sattva*' leads to the fifth stage which is *decrease in worldly attractions.*
6. Decrease in worldly attractions leads to the sixth stage which is *giving up of worldly objects.*
7. Giving up of worldly objects leads to the seventh and the final stage, which is *freedom from all thoughts about one's own self and its consequential benefits.*

Once I saw a Mahatma at Amarkantak, who wore no clothes at all. I asked him why he was breaking the universally accepted social custom of covering the body, and what was wrong with it. However, I saw that when he felt thirsty he did not ask for water by word of the mouth but only *looked* thirsty. Someone gave him a glass of water. Although he drank it, he did not even hold the glass in his hand. This showed how he resorted to no physical action to satisfy his bodily needs. This was his own way of leading a free life. Of course he could have done it a little differently!

Questions of procedure should be answered in the language of procedure. Questions relating to prayer should be answered in the language of prayer. Those relating to *Vedanta* should be answered in the language of *Vedanta*. Otherwise they would amount to offering something which is not actually needed – like offering food to one who is not hungry, or water to one who is not thirsty. As regards the method of approach through prayer, here, procedural errors can be forgiven. But this is not an ideal, nor even a rule.

Observance of the various disciplines alone does not get us up to the *Param-Atman;* it only purifies the *Chitta*, and then *Param-Atman* Himself comes into it. The observance of disciplines is necessary only until the melting and purification of *Chitta* is complete.

These ideas do not arise in thinkers. Thinkers actually want nothing, not even God. *(See page 121)* They only want a purification of the *Antahkarana*.

Finally, may I mention that though *Prarabdha* can be helpful or unhelpful in our worldly efforts, yet it would not stand in the way of our spiritual progress. For example, recitation of a Mantra would be useful even if the back is not straight. If circumstances do not let us sit down to worship in the prescribed manner, we can do it mentally in any way the circumstances permit. But what is wrong is to postpone it. Postponing a debt does not save us from repaying it, but only increases the burden of interest we have to pay in the end.

29 January
Mela Talk

The previous speaker explained the story of Sita, the wife of Rama, as unfolded for us in the epic *Ramayana*. Just as King Rama represents the fundamental *Param-Atman*, similarly Sita, his queen, represents fundamental energy. Energy is the capacity of a body to perform work. A bodiless *Param-Atman* can therefore perform no work and it has to adopt energy for this purpose. But if energy is adopted, there should be some identity to adopt it – otherwise there can be no adoption. If there is to be any energy, there should also be a vehicle to convey it; just as if there are waves there should also be a medium for them.

The two identities of the fundamental *Param-Atman* and the fundamental energy, though going by separate names and allotted different attributes as a matter of convenience, are intrinsically inseparable from each other. Thus Rama and Sita, though different, are yet the same. And all that is attributed to Rama in the story of Rama and Sita, is done by Sita because, without energy, work cannot be done.

Actually, it is only the display of energy that can introduce us to the possessor of energy – the *Param-Atman*. Thus energy attracts us towards the presence of *Param-Atman*. That is what goes in the *Upanishads* by the name of *Brahma-Vidya*, the Divine Knowledge.

People possessing knowledge sometimes become too much obsessed with it and begin to feel a pride of superiority, even condemning *Bhakti* (devotional way). This is misuse of knowledge. Pride, too, has a place in our lives and we may all possess it, but of course using it only to prevent ourselves from stooping low into undignified tendencies. So also has the individual ego (*Ahankara*) a place in our lives and its use is that of an incentive to duty. For example, the *Ahankar* of being a policeman should impel a policeman to perform his duties with all the dignity of his rank.

It is the 'Department of the Interior' (Autonomic) which sends us towards the path of *Bhakti*. *Bhakti* has more use for ideology than for any intellectual reasoning. For one on the path of *Bhakti*, even if the judgement goes wrong at times over details, then frequently it does not matter.

We make much of our human intellect, the *Buddhi*. But we forget that it is designed to work only within worldly limits. *Param-Atman* is beyond the worldly limits and hence out of reach of the *Buddhi*. Here a devoted heart reaches the goal. *Buddhi* can, at the utmost, carry us up to the door and then it must leave us there to take care of ourselves, having itself no further access. As it cannot go further, all it can do then is to keep us away from *Param-Atman*.

In the context of *Bhakti*, the example of Kunti (the bereaved mother in the *Mahabharata* epic) furnishes an interesting argument. It is unique in the sense that no one but her has ever asked specifically to be given adversities, whereas everyone else throughout history has asked for deliverance from adversities.

> When Krishna was leaving after the war, all others asked for this or that favour. When the turn of Kunti came, she said, 'Give me some adversity or other to remain with me all the time.'
> 'But why adversity?'
> 'Because in the past I always thought of You and brought You near me whenever there was adversity, and never when there was none.'

3 February
Mela Talk

Wisdom lives in the heart of all of us, but instead of flowing as a constant stream, it flows and ebbs intermittently. This is why we act sometimes rightly and sometimes wrongly; sometimes we are virtuous, sometimes sinful. Every year you assemble here for the *Mela*, and no doubt you benefit from the contact and preaching of the Holy men you find here. But this effect does not last, and by the time of the next *Mela* many of you may lose what you gain and become as you were before. Then you attend another *Mela*, gain something only to lose it again. So this alternate gain and loss goes on indefinitely, each neutralising the other and your remaining days of life becoming fewer and fewer. Even during your ordinary life wisdom shines and fades intermittently. We are very holy at times, and very unholy at times; sometimes we dream of having become a king, sometimes of being reduced to beggary. The reason for all this is that we have pushed *Param-Atman* into the background and kept *Ahankara* in the foreground.

The word '*Ahankara*' is frequently treated as a synonym for pride in ordinary language, and we consider it as an undesirable quality. If you have any *Ahankara* at all, better raise it sky-high, otherwise let it go down, down, down.

> A Mahatma used to say, 'There is no Mahatma like me.' People said, 'It is the limit of *Ahankara* to say so. How does it behove you, who are a Mahatma?' He replied, 'Everyone else is either better than me, or worse. But none is exactly the same as I, so I am right.'

This has a deeper meaning. Indeed, everyone of us is unique, having no equal anywhere in the world. Still, it has become fashionable nowadays to talk of equality. But how can you find equality *anywhere* in the vast field of creation? The world exhibits nothing but variety, and variety means nothing but the existence of differences. If these differences, the differences between one thing and another, disappear, then the whole world would disappear, as it does in a state of dreamless sleep.

You just now heard the story of how Hanuman burnt down Lanka, the fortress of Ravana. Our physical bodies are like the Lanka, the fortress of evil. Let us 'burn' it with the fire of wisdom. The Lanka, having been thus burned, the *Ahankara* living in it will also burn off. Then there would be nothing left to hide the *Param-Atman*.

Instead of doing this, people invariably go and ask a Mahatma or a Guru, 'Sir, be gracious enough to show me the *Param-Atman*. I am very anxious for that'. But the poor Guru has to do a tremendous amount of spadework before he can do that, for which people have no patience.

> For example, the Prince of Tehri once met Swami Ram Tirtha and asked him, 'Swami Ji, can you show God to me?'
>
> 'Yes. But before I do that, can you tell me exactly what you are? Are you the body I see, or something else?'
>
> 'Oh! Not exactly.'
>
> 'Well, when you are so ignorant that you do not know even who you are, who can show you the great God?'

3 February
Ashram Talk

Two kinds of forces live in all of us – good and evil. Their co-existence leads to conflict, and conflict leads to unhappiness. Had there been no such conflict, there would have been a perpetual state of happiness. Forces of evil like desire, anger, etc., exist in saints also, but the difference is that they do good to others instead of harming them. Liberation implies freeing the *Chitta* from this duality of good and evil.

The universe also unfolds itself in two ways. One way is the way of '*Avidya*', ignorance, in which we imagine ourselves to be the 'doers' of actions, and are, therefore, subject to the law of 'Karma', that is, 'as you sow, so you reap'. The other way is like the performance of a drama, in which the actor acting as a thief or a saint, is not a thief or a saint. In this, therefore, the law of 'Karma' does not hold.

For example: In cases where *Param-Atman* took the part of a man according to Hindu Scriptures, He was not really a man. Thus he was not bound by the 'Karmas' He performed as such.

This cannot be the case with a person who identifies himself with his actions. If anyone *thinks* that he has won a victory today, the Law of *Karma* lays down that he would suffer a defeat tomorrow.

It is said that when evils are absent, we meet *Param-Atman*. This may not always be true. For example, a tree has no evils, and yet we cannot say that it has met *Param-Atman*. A pitcher with its mouth turned downwards will never get filled with water even if it rains heavily.

Similarly, *Param-Atman* is pouring His favours on us constantly, but we do not benefit from it as we are turned away from Him. *Param-Atman* tries to help us all the time, but it is our own help that is lacking.

It takes nine months for a human embryo to develop into a baby, but it takes only an instant to die. Similarly, the cumulative effect of years of practice can be nullified in minutes.

An old woman lived in a village. It was winter and a cat died in her home. She thought that if she threw it away in the daytime, she would have to take a bath afterwards as otherwise her neighbours would regard her as unclean. So she waited till night. When everybody was fast asleep, she quietly went to the river a little distance away and threw it into the water.

By the time she got back home, a sick camel had strayed into her courtyard and died there. Now the carcass needed several strong men to drag it out. Therefore the whole village came to know of it and the old woman could not avoid a bath.

Something similar applies to renunciation and involvement.

A bondage is a bondage after all. It does not matter whether it is a golden chain that binds you, or one of iron. Of course, the golden chain is attractive, but a prisoner is a prisoner, whether he is awarded an 'A' class, or a 'B' class, or a 'C' class in the prison. Worldly pleasures are like 'A' class accommodation in a prison, and troubles like 'C' class.

4 February
Ashram Talk

What is (the) world? What is Truth? What are you? Well, we want to find out all that. You are '*Sat-Chit-Ananda*', that is, eternal reality, full of power and joy, etc. But how? Just think whether you have any personal knowledge as to how and when you were born. You only know the date and time of your birth as you have heard from others. You never actually experienced your birth. Then take it that you were never born, and a thing which is not born cannot die either. Thus, you are unborn and deathless, and so are '*Sat-Chit-Ananda*'.

Ravana is a Sanskrit name. It means, 'one who makes you sleep'. It is said that he had ten heads. Then, how could he go to sleep with ten heads? Just as we do. The ten heads were imaginary or metaphorical. You are also a 'Ravana'. Your 'ten heads' are the ten organs of action and senses. Ravana's fortress is said to have been made of gold, Lanka. The Sanskrit word for gold has two meanings, that is, the noun '*gold*' and the verb '*to sleep*'. Gold attracts and so did Lanka; Lanka was devoid of True Knowledge so it was 'sleeping'.

'*Satsanga*' is good company. We get it through the company of Holy books, through the company of Holy men, and through the company of *Param-Atman*. In order that we do not get confused and lost in a labyrinth of ideas, all these 'companions' are necessary, otherwise it is like treating yourself for a disease by reading medical books, or something similar.

> A frog sat beneath a lotus flower. Instead of enjoying its sweet fragrance, it only ate dirty worms from the mud below. A beetle knew what was good in a lotus, it sat over it and enjoyed the fragrance.

If we give some time to reading Holy books, some time to thinking of *Param-Atman*, then our wisdom matures; darkness no longer frightens us, and we attain supreme happiness. Not only so, but we begin to radiate happiness which affects the surroundings as well as those around us, be they men, birds or animals.

> The story goes that a mere dog got rid of its wretchedness by the company of Yudhishthira.

But if we do not practice *Satsanga* in the above manner, then the thought of *Param-Atman* recedes to the background and *Ahankara* comes to the fore. Ignorant worldly people, however, see no sense in all this and treat it as a waste of time.

> One, Shri Malviya, used to meditate on *Param-Atman* for two hours daily. One of his friends said, 'why do you sit idle for two hours each day? Instead of wasting them in this manner, you could do some work to benefit yourself or somebody else.'
>
> He replied, 'All right, I am wasting two hours, but you are wasting twenty-two hours!'

9 February
Ashram Talk

All living beings seem to be crying out for something or other. Among mankind some pray for wealth, some for health, some for property, some for fame, some for power, some for freedom from troubles, some for food and basic necessities during life. Moreover, all want what they ask for to be on a permanent basis; nobody wants a merely temporary cure or temporary riches. Also, we want these things in full measure, and nothing which is less than full is good enough, our object being to make ourselves full in all respects.

The Scriptures belonging to every religion devote thought to the question of what among all these things is really worth praying for. If we study those Scriptures accessible to us, it would seem as if all of them want *Param- Atman*, because it is *He* only who is completely full in all respects and His fullness can never decrease. All the rest are neither full nor permanent. Thus, people seem really to be wanting the *Param-Atman* though they do not realise this.

Ravana (in the epic *Ramayana*, the enemy of King Rama) had a big kingdom, a big family, a big palace, a big army, a big treasury, and everything. Everybody looked at him with awe and reverence, ready to carry out his commands. And yet, not only was he not at peace, but even a time came when he lost all and nothing remained.

When one is a child, one wants toys; when one is a boy, one wants education; when one's education is over, one wants employment; when one gets employment, one wants promotion. Thus, from the beginning to the very end, there is never contentment.

> The great Moghul Emperor Akbar, while out hunting, once had to spend the night in the jungle. Unable to sleep owing to the noise made by jackals, he asked why they were crying. Someone said that it was on account of the cold. Akbar ordered blankets to be distributed to the jackals, but still they went on crying. When Akbar again asked the reason, he was told that it was on account of their joy at getting the blankets.

In this way satisfaction never comes to us, and we always go on crying!

The remedy is devoting yourself to *Param-Atman*. With this, all the unnecessary thinking of worldly needs comes to an end, and thereafter is succeeded by Realisation of *Param-Atman*. Only then is there complete satisfaction, wanting nothing we feel full. A union takes place between the full Self and the full *Param-Atman*. These two aspects of fullness mingle inseparably, never to part again.

Though *Param-Atman* manifests Himself in everything, everything suffers some kind of pollution, yet *Param-Atman* Himself always remains unpolluted, just as gold remains gold, even after being shaped and reshaped a thousand times into various ornaments. As long as we do not know *Param-Atman*, our belief in Him remains half-hearted, only when we know Him does our belief become firm and unshakable.

10 February
Ashram Talk

If we do not see *Param-Atman* everywhere in the vast field of creation, and do not see its sweetness, and are not filled with joy by it, then we really see nothing at all. Then our practice lacks in weight.

So *Param-Atman* is in everything. Let your heart be filled with joy on seeing how *Param-Atman* manifests in everything. Then if *Param-Atman* lives in your whole vision, He also lives in your heart.

A housewife stood at her door looking her best in an attractive costume and makeup waiting to receive her husband back home from work.

A Mahatma passed that way, and he fixed his eyes on her. There was a volley of protests that a Mahatma should be the last person to stare at women; some even threatened to lynch him.

The Mahatma said, 'I am only admiring the art and the beauty of God's creation. I have nothing to do with you, who call yourselves men or women though you are made of the same flesh and blood in each case.' And he walked away.

Indeed, despite all the visible differences, there are more similarities than dissimilarities between men and women. A story illustrates the point:

> A woman managed to sneak into the male police force. She put in long years of service undetected, performing her duties creditably. But when retiring, she revealed the truth. Everyone was surprised, and she was rewarded for faithful service instead of being prosecuted for impersonation.

There are two kinds of worlds, soft and hard. Similarly, there are men, soft and hard. Those who are soft in nature will benefit from belief while those who are hard in nature will benefit from thought. Believers would ordinarily shun thinkers, and *vice versa*. But both can attain fullness, and if they can be brought to coexistence in a group, they are good for each other.

Someone argued that Sannyasins shunned work and were therefore dead people for all practical purposes. But *really* dead is the one who considers himself to be only the physical body, which is mortal and full of ignorance, and not the one who considers himself to be the *Atman*, which is immortal and full of knowledge.

The path to *Param-Atman* via Knowledge is beset with many obstacles, which are such that only a few can get through. Even when major progress has been made, the greatest risk comes towards the end where *Maya* tries to beguile us. If we begin to falter at that stage, then a downfall takes place which undoes everything. Pleasant impediments, being of a tempting nature, are actually far more dangerous than the unpleasant ones, because the former possess more appeal than the latter. It is attachment to worldly things which is the root of all troubles.

Either you accept *Param-Atman* first and then proceed to know Him, or you try something first and then accept. The important thing is confidence and not effort. If you go on living in the present, then the past and the future would take care of themselves.

For raising the level of thought, thinking of *Param-Atman* is the right thing. If you think that everything is *Param-Atman*, then love deepens. But if love decreases, we fall. Actually, it is love which is our greatest asset.

12 February
Ashram Talk

For controlling the flood of a river, we have to do two things: build a dam and dig out a canal. A canal reduces the volume of water in the main stream, making control easy. Similarly, for controlling our thoughts, let us divert some of them towards a Holy direction, and let us raise an obstruction towards the unholy direction. Holy thoughts often take us to the company of Holy men. This, in turn, creates in us an objective judgement, which is helpful in realising *Param-Atman*. But in fact, Holy company is most difficult to find in the materialistic world of today. If we are lucky enough to get it, then our *Chitta* becomes absorbed in it, and then reaching *Param-Atman* does not remain difficult. So Holy thoughts and actions do not by themselves carry us direct to *Param-Atman*, but they can take us to Holy company which, in turn, leads us to *Param-Atman*.

The specialty of human birth is the possession of a pure judgement. This, if taken advantage of, takes us to Holy company, and there we find the key which unlocks all secrets. It frequently happens that if one secret is unlocked, the unlocking of others follows. In the eyes of thinking men, liberation and bondage are merely a drama. Actually, none is in bondage. Had there been a real bondage, it would not have been possible to undo it. We only think we are under bondage, and liberation only means removal of this thought. Birth and death are also a drama; nobody can experience his own birth or death; we can only hear about it from others, whereas statements of others can always differ and therefore cannot be regarded as true.

We go on criticising and criticising, little realising that criticism demolishes much and builds little. Our powers of reasoning also disprove more and prove less, even on the worldly plane. But *Param-Atman* is beyond human reasoning. You cannot advance sufficient reasons to satisfy everybody about even the existence of *Param-Atman*, not to speak of reaching Him, through reasoning alone. What we can do is to cleanse the heart, then He shows Himself up on His own accord.

15 February
Questions from FCR

HH: You want to know that, from all the discourses you have had with me so far, what exactly is the most important for you today. My difficulty is that, unless I can recall all you asked and all I said in reply, I cannot be in a position to say that. Roughly, however, it may suffice to indicate that the gist of all that should be:

1. Physically, you devote yourself to universal service, considering yourself everyone's servant.

2. Devotionally, you give importance to the Supreme Power, keeping in mind its unlimited benevolence.

3. Intellectually, you identify yourSelf as one with *Param-Atman*, who witnesses everything and shows Himself in all the forms you see.

You say, 'It seems impossible to give it all up just yet, but I can keep it usually to only two days a week. . .'

Now, 'giving up' can be done emotionally and intellectually at all times and in all conditions. In this, there is no question of today or tomorrow, or of one or two days a week. Practise 'giving up' all the time. You just consider the body, the heart and the mind as belonging to *Param-Atman* and as such, offer all these back to *Param-Atman*. That is what 'giving up' means.

You seem to ask how to maintain Sattva.

If *Rajas* and *Tamas* arise during the prevalence of *Sattva*, then they would be ineffective. For this, you should off and on recall the idea of your real Self, and at the same time keep yourself engaged in doing service (which is your duty). Then, because of *Sattva* intervening between *Rajas* and *Tamas*, the latter would not notably affect your *Antahkarana*. A little *Sattva* will cure much *Rajas* and *Tamas*, just as a small quantity of medicine cures a big disease. Or, say, just as a little matchstick can burn down a mountain of cotton.

15 February
Ashram Talk

No worldly action, however good, can be entirely free from evil.
No worldly pleasure can be obtained without causing pain to
someone. Every sinner has a virtue. Should we, then, abstain
from action in order to get away from evil?

The way to rid oneself from evil is to cultivate the attitude that it
is nature that is acting through the body, and not the Self. The
body is the machine of nature to produce action. Your Self is only
the witness, and not the doer. It is through nature that *Param-
Atman* is making the whole universe dance, but He does not dance
Himself. He makes our *Manas*, *Buddhi*, etc., dance, but none can
make Him dance. He is the Reality and the Truth, and there is no
place where He is lacking. The states of *Chitta* are not the states of
Atman. Meditation, practice, *Samadhi*, etc., are all states of *Chitta*.

Even digging the ground for the service of *Param-Atman* is
heavenly, while worship of *Param-Atman* for worldly ends is
hellish. For practising remembrance of *Param-Atman*, do not wait
for a suitable opportunity. Do not think of today or tomorrow.
You can do it whenever a feeling of devotion arises in your heart,
paying no heed to the hindrances present.

> This is how a doctor got over his hindrances. He had an
> ill-tempered wife. He got a telephone call to see a patient
> at eight o'clock one night. The wife said that dinner
> would be ready at nine o'clock, and that he could have it
> when he got back. The doctor said that he would be back
> by then. But he was held up until midnight, when the
> wife had gone to bed and the dinner had got cold. On
> hearing the horn of his car, the wife woke up and started

116

nagging the doctor. He put the dinner on her head.
'What do you mean?' she asked with double anger. 'I am
heating my dinner. It has got cold,' answered the doctor.

Someone asked a Mahatma the way to get to the *Param-Atman*. The Mahatma told him to run.

'Is running the way to *Param-Atman*?'

'Maybe, but not the only way.'

Similarly, remembering the *Param-Atman* can be one way, but not the only way. No one way can be universal.

16 February
Ashram Talk

This talk continues the same theme as His Holiness's discourse on 9 February, and shows that only after becoming acquainted could one become a devotee:

Normally it should be the incomplete who would seek the complete. Therefore, one who is already complete should have no necessity to seek the complete. But, strangely, it is only the completed Being that would seek the complete *Param-Atman*. It is so because it can only be the completed Self which would automatically go into the thought of *Param-Atman* as soon as it sits down quietly. As long as anything else can attract you, be sure that *Param-Atman* is far away. After all, you cannot ride two horses at the same time.

As *Param-Atman* is all-powerful and limitless, it is obvious that no bondage could tie Him. But it is strange, again, that strings of love and *Bhakti* can do so. We know that only acquaintance can create love. *Param-Atman* is so beautiful that the more we get acquainted with Him, the more we get filled with joy. This creates *Bhakti* automatically and necessarily. Then, acts of worship become redundant. They do, however, constitute a preliminary necessity.

It should be understood here that that so-called 'devotion' (which we can attempt before acquaintance) is a forced phenomenon and unreal, while that which sets in, after acquaintance, is real. Then our body, mind and all possessions become dedicated to *Param-Atman*, and this dedication itself becomes the worship of *Param-Atman*. Then we eat, drink, act, etc., for the sake of *Param-Atman* and do nothing for ourselves. Everywhere and in everything we see nothing but *Param-Atman*. This is a stage of absolute intimacy with *Param-Atman*, and *Bhakti* is just another word for this stage.

Now, let us revert to the question of acquaintance once again. Without being acquainted with a thing, any love or worship offered to it would be insincere. The question therefore is, how to acquire this acquaintance. Worldly acquaintances can be got by trying. But *Param-Atman* is outside the worldly sphere. So human trials to catch Him all fail, unless and until He Himself comes within our grip. This He does as soon as He sees that we deserve it. So, what we should do is to deserve it.

Holy company provides us with a training ground for all this. One of the things we learn from it is that the deepest possible relationship that can exist between two things is that which exists between our Self and *Param-Atman*. All other relationships are less. A realisation of this fact can give a lot of *Bhakti*, and we reach our goal.

22 February
Ashram Talk

As compared with the lower animals, the development of power is more marked in the human being. This power resides in the *Antahkarana*.

Now take the case of an electric bulb. We generally see that a bigger bulb is more powerful in respect of giving light. Therefore a question arises: what is it that should matter – the size of the bulb or the light it gives? If the bulb is blue, the light appears to be blue; if it is red, the light appears red; if it is clear, the light appears clear; if it is dirty, the light appears dirty. In spite of all this the light itself was the same in each case. It was intrinsically neither blue, nor red, nor dirty.

Just as the differences were created by the bulb while the light remained the same, similarly the differences in power displayed by men is created by the *Antahkarana*, while *Param-Atman*, the source of power, remains always the same. From poets the same power expresses itself as poetry, from scientists as science, from lawyers as law, from soldiers as soldiery, from athletes as athletics, etc. Some manifest the power more and some less, but the power itself is neither more nor less from case to case.

Certain things are considered pure and others impure; but *Param-Atman*, the basis of all, is One and the same. Then, how does purity and impurity come in? The reason lies in the two phases of power – '*Vidya*' and '*Avidya*' (knowledge and ignorance). This, in turn, gives rise to two kinds of nature in creation, pure and impure. And, all the time, there is a process going on tending to set right the things that have gone wrong owing to *Avidya*.

If a pot goes out of shape, the potter would undo it and make it again. If part of a machine does not come up to the correct specifications, the factory recasts it as required. The material does not become useless, but is used again to produce the correct article. Wrong things are being constantly turned into right things.

All these corrective processes are going on in Nature, not in *Param-Atman*. After all, nature is just another word for behaviour.

Nature is not free to act independently. The power puts up various shows to please its Master. Nature, owing to her subordinate relationship with *Param-Atman*, wants to win His favour. This can only be done by producing things which He can like, and only the rightly produced things would be liked.

Our hands, feet, eyes, ears, etc., are intended by Nature to act correctly, so that *Param-Atman* may be pleased, but owing to ignorance, we believe that they are meant to please the world!

Though *Param-Atman* is limitless, yet we have to see Him first in limited things. Seeing Him in limited things would eventually lead us to the unlimited *Param-Atman*. The inertness of the *Chitta* stands in the way of realising Him. Love has the power to remove this inertness and give us a glimpse of *Param-Atman*.

12 April
Discourse by His Holiness

Antahkarana
You are right in saying that it is an 'inner organ' or cell, and that it is not physical in the sense that it can be seen. From this *Antahkarana*, light is felt in the shape of *Ahankara*, *Buddhi*, and

Manas. It is dealt with at length in books on Indian philosophy. Its influence is particularly seen in the waking and dreaming states. During dreamless sleep, it is quiet. In the *Turiya* state, it is lacking.

Thinkers want nothing; not even God
This means that they realise that everything belongs to *Param-Atman* and is inseparably related to Him. Therefore there is no dearth of anything for them. When there is no dearth, the question of needing or wanting would not arise. Those who are surrounded with needs and wants, they, in reality, do not want the *Param-Atman* but the fulfilment of their wants and needs through Him. Such a person has neither love nor knowledge.

Making a friend of Buddhi
Buddhi always tries to follow the *Atman*. *Manas* is its child; but when *Manas* begins to pull and attract it, then it deviates from its Master and bends towards the *Manas*, and the *Manas* follows external pleasures.

Therefore, when *Buddhi* is free to love the *Atman*, and *Manas* follows *Buddhi*, deficiency vanishes and sufficiency reigns supreme in which nothing can be lacking.

29 April
Ashram Talk

Love is the active force behind all the processes at work in the world to sustain it. There could be no sustenance unless some feeling of love exists. In the case of the human life, its examples are the love of parents, the love of brothers, the love of friends and colleagues, etc. Even the behaviour of insects and moths seems to be based on some form of love. So much so, that the ultimate cause of hostility is also love. Because hostility springs up when love is hindered. Thus a duality of love and hostility prevails everywhere. We want a thing that we love; if we do not get it we turn hostile.

A love free from the above duality is true love. Love for a thing which is not there is deception. The whole drama enacted by *Param-Atman* depicts this one thing only. But there is none to understand it.

As it were, a perennial game of hide-and-seek seems to be going on. We are all seeking something. Some seek it in annihilation, some in creation, some in light, some in darkness, some in intellect, etc. Actually it is *Param-Atman* that all are seeking, and *Param-Atman* is hidden in all these things and in everything else. But, while seeking, people have forgotten what actually they *are* seeking.

> A man wanted to go to his father-in-law's place to meet his wife. He went to the railway station where the train was just about to leave, and he shouted at the booking clerk, 'A ticket to my father-in-law's place, please.'
>
> 'Name of place, please,' quipped the booking clerk.'
>
> 'Oh, my father-in-law's place! Please! Please! Now! Quickly!'
>
> 'But why won't you tell me the name of the place?'
>
> 'I'm telling you! My father-in-law's place! For God's sake, quick! The train is about to start.' And the train started leaving the man behind.
>
> Something like that is happening to all of us.

Ramana Maharshi went on meditating for fourteen years over the question, 'Who am I?'. As soon as he was on the right path, it took him only a minute to realise that he was everything.

When Rama was searching for Sita in the forests, he was so much lost in his thoughts that he forgot everything about himself. He asked such questions from Lakshman, 'Who am I? What is this? What is that? Where am I? How did I get here?'

When Lakshman reminded him, he recovered his wits but soon lapsed back into senselessness again. Over and over these questions were asked and answered, but forgotten again and again.

This is what is happening with all of us. In a state of perpetual senselessness, we have been searching for something without finding it. We want to know what we are. We want to be happy. That is, we are seeking *Param-Atman*. But *Param-Atman* is sitting in everything, though there is a curtain of ignorance between Him and us.

We should see *Param-Atman* in everything. If we do that, we receive special favours from Him. Then this curtain of ignorance lifts up and the *Maya*, which has been cheating us all the time, no longer does so and begins to help us instead.

January 1973
Discourse by His Holiness

His Holiness was speaking about the *four ways*, beginning with the three Traditional Ways, those of the *man of action*, the *knowledge seeker*, and the *devotee*. He said that they can all be motivated by some personal ambition or desire, so that people would always lay claim to the results of their desires and ambitions.'

That refers to the Traditional Ways, all of which are some variant of these three – the way of action, the way of knowledge and the way of devotion.

HH: What the first Shri Shankara stressed in starting the great *Advaita* System or Tradition of non-duality, was the necessity to remove that desire, that ambition, and those claims, so that through all the different ways the will of the Absolute could be fulfilled. After all, the will of the Absolute is perfect, needing no modification, so why bother to have any other desires but to fulfil that will? To have no personal desire is to *accept* the will of the Absolute. Having established this, one could fulfil a complete life.

> There was once an elephant, a king of elephants, who was large and mighty and proud of it! Once, when he went to the river for a bathe and a drink, he was caught by a crocodile who dragged him into deep water where the elephant had nothing to hold on to. All his struggles were in vain. When he was almost drowned, he reached out with the tip of his trunk and picked up a floating flower, and, offering it to the Lord, he prayed for compassion and release. The prayer was truly sincere, and the Lord responded by running fast and smiting the crocodile. So the elephant was rescued and came out of the river.
>
> Suddenly he saw a luminous body moving towards the high heaven, so he asked the Lord what it was. He was told that it was the crocodile on his way to heaven. The elephant found this surprising, for was it not he who had called to God for help, and now God was taking his sinful aggressor up to heaven. He begged for an explanation.

God said, 'You called me with an exclusive desire to save yourself, a desire which was fulfilled. But in the fulfilling of your desire, the crocodile was killed for no very good reason. He had to receive compensation therefore, and this has now been arranged.'

The way of action, knowledge, or even devotion, when accompanied with personal desire or ambition is limited to the desire. Undo the desire and it becomes unlimited.

APPENDIX

Bhakti

Question from FCR (September 1975)

HH has been quoted as saying: 'For different ends there are different means: for Liberation, Knowledge; for Power, Yoga; for *Param-Atman, Bhakti*. A *Bhakta* is already liberated, otherwise he could not get started. He is not troubled about either Heaven or Hell. He would be quite content with Hell if he found *Param-Atman* there.' This saying has suddenly seemed illuminating and important to me, but I want to be sure we are not misquoting His Holiness. It appeals to both my heart and my mind!

HH: The incentive is that God is certainly available to everyone everywhere and in the most simple way, but the simplicity has been lost so people are separated. Not that they are in reality separated, but they *feel* separated, because they have forgotten the union. It is forgetfulness which comes between the *Param-Atman* and the individual. Otherwise the *Param-Atman* is simply available to everyone who desires him.

As far as *Bhakti* is concerned the observation made is true and right because whenever anyone goes on the way of *Bhakti* or devotion, then it seems he is not bothered about anything else except the *Param-Atman*, so it does not matter where he is, what he is facing, whatever the situation or the time – he is not concerned – so whether it is Heaven, or Hell or anything else, if he feels he is united with the *Param-Atman* it would not matter – all are equally good.

The same is said by Tulsi Das in his *Ramayana*. Tulsi Das says that Heaven, Hell and Liberation are all just the same thing for him because he sees Rama everywhere holding his bow and arrows (the symbols of Rama), and Tulsi Das sees him everywhere, wherever he lifts his eyes.

The *Muni* ('sage' or literally, 'the mute one'), or man of Knowledge, is equally similar to the *Bhakta*. As quoted in the scriptures, whatever the man of knowledge studies, whatever he analyses, he is only looking at the finer aspects of the *Param-Atman*. If he is doing that, he is the real wise man; if he does not see this in his enquiry, then he is looking for something else. So the language of the *Bhakta* and of the *Muni* or wise man is almost identical, and they both speak a universal language; they rarely refer to the particular, or to the individual.

In the *Gita*, the same thing is mentioned again and again, and it says that out of the four types one is the *Arta* type – the one who cries for the Lord. So one can acquire union with the *Param-Atman*, apart from anything else, just by crying, if that is the ultimate end of one's crying.

> A Mahatma was approached by an ordinary man and asked what he should do – he did not feel he could undergo much discipline so what was the simplest form? The Mahatma said he could find *Param-Atman* by running.
>
> The man asked, 'If *Param-Atman* can be found by running, why not just by sitting?' Yes' he replied, 'perhaps also by sitting, but the question is, what are you sitting *for*? If you are sitting for the *Param-Atman*, *Param-Atman* will meet you, if you are running for the *Param-Atman*, *Param-Atman* will meet you there also. You can do anything, it does not really matter – the real crux is whether you are doing it for *Param-Atman*, for the sake of *Param-Atman*, or for something of this world.' The Mahatma continued by

saying that the Unity is already there, nobody has to acquire it, but because we have all forgotten our unity, we are only required to give up our ignorance, give up our forgetfulness by any means that we can.

All these Yogas; *Raja* Yoga, *Ashtanga* Yoga etc., are all leading towards only one aspect, that the individual who wants to go by any of these ways has to decide once and for all that whatever he does, he does it for the *Param-Atman*, and then he will find this union.

If you try to do anything, just to fulfil your worldly desires and commitments – however gloriously you may function – then you will find that the union which is already there will not be experienced. The thing to decide is that one is doing everything for the *Param-Atman* – even digging the earth, or anything at all one likes to do.

In the *Gita* it says that people should take to this through their own vocation, whatever they are destined to do (in fact, whatever they may find themselves doing is good enough) and that is their way, that is their Yoga for unity with the *Param-Atman*. The only important thing is that everything must be done for the *Param-Atman*, and nothing should be done to acquire any particular object except union with the *Param-Atman*.

One should just surrender oneself and the feeling of surrender itself is the gate of liberation. A *Bhakta* is always liberated because he is not bothered about anything except the *Param-Atman*; and when only this one idea, the *Param-Atman*, reigns in the mind, then that is liberation. A *Bhakta* does not necessarily undertake any particular discipline; he simply lives a liberated life.

The Gunas *(August 1979)*

HH: The Law of Three prevails at every stage and is involved in every event of life. There is nothing which escapes the Law of Three. The Law of Three was previously discussed as physical, subtle and causal and also as *Tamasic, Rajasic* and *Sattvic*. Whatever event you like to see and visualise or analyse you will find the Law of Three at work. In relation to the *Ahankar*, each individual who has a unified concept of himself and a picture evolving out of this unified concept of the world, as he sees it, the way he behaves is governed by this Law of Three. If the person is *Tamasic* then he sees himself within *Tamas* and is seen to be composed mostly of *Tamasic* elements. He will see the world in a *Tamasic* way. Similarly, *Rajasic* or *Sattvic*.

The same can be seen in *Bhajana*[†] – the devotional activity which disciples or householders take up. In *Tamasic Bhajana* sometimes people engage themselves in a peculiar discipline of controlling the evil forces, ghosts and the like, they perform certain rituals and keep on doing this for a long time so that they may acquire the possibility of dictating their desires to these evil forces who would respond so that their desires may be fulfilled.

The *Rajasic* type of *Bhajana,* or devotion, is mostly related to different levels of gods. There is a variety of gods in a hierarchy under the *Param-Atman* and some people engage themselves in pleasing these gods by devotional acts and continued practices of rituals and when they have finally pleased them and they have acquired their favour everything that happens to them is favourable and their desires are fulfilled.

The man who goes on the way of *Sattvic Bhajana,* he attends only to the *Param-Atman*. He does not have any particular desire to be fulfilled, he devotes himself simply without desire. Accordingly he

---

[†]Bhajana: *Yoga Vedanta Dictionary* = Worship and praise of the Lord. Taking refuge in the Lord.

will acquire great powers. He does not look for results and he does not have any particular desires. These are the three ways showing the Law of Three working through the *Bhajana* or devotion.

We can see the same thing in relation to thought, action and sleep. A really healthy man needs only a few hours of sleep and after that he should be happy and strong enough to perform all sorts of vigorous physical or intellectual work. *Tamasic* people keep on sleeping for hour after hour, eight or ten hours and even after that they are not very happy to get out of their beds. They keep on desiring more sleep. It never gives them any proper rest and never gives them any more power but in this way they waste their lives in sloth.

Rajasic sleep is when you keep on having all sorts of worries in your mind and keep on dreaming or creating dreams, or weaving desires and plans for achievements. You waste the whole time that you intend to rest and you never get any proper sleep and again engage yourself in further activity.

In *Sattvic* sleep you would immediately go to sleep the moment you are in bed and after a few hours you are fully refreshed and awake so that you can attend to everything that is necessary.

There we have the Law of Three related to the being, the attitude of an individual through which he activates himself in relation to the world. Again, in relation to *Samadhi* the Law of Three prevails.

There was a man who had trained himself in physical *Samadhi*. He went to a king who owned a black horse that he coveted. He said to the king that he would demonstrate his *Samadhi*, lasting twelve years, and as a reward for this exemplary *Samadhi* he would like to be given the black horse from the king's stables. The king agreed and all the necessary arrangements for his *Samadhi* were made. A trench was dug, he was placed in it and covered with planks and soil. Then everybody forgot about him. Sometime during these twelve years the king died and so did the horse. The desire of the man in *Samadhi* remained alive because he was neither asleep nor dead, he was in *Samadhi*.

After twelve years the situation in the kingdom had changed completely. Some people were building a new palace at the *Samadhi* site. When they came across the man in *Samadhi* they dug him out. When he returned to consciousness he asked for his black horse. What black horse, they asked? He said, well, where is the king? Can you call him? They said the king had died. He explained that the old king had agreed to give him his black horse after twelve years of *Samadhi*, which he had now completed. Could he please now have the horse? Then they told him that the black horse was also dead and consequently he could now have nothing.

This is an example of *Tamasic Samadhi*, as there was something which he wanted to acquire after twelve years of non-activity – non-productive *Samadhi*.

There is also *Rajasic Samadhi*, when you get peace after doing some activity. After a little peace you once again rush into activity and keep on with this cycle of activity and peace. It keeps you going but it does not improve the situation though, of course, there may not be any loss either.

As an example of *Sattvic Samadhi* there is the *Rasaleela*. As a youth, the Lord Krishna used to dance with the *Gopi* girls in the jungles of Mathura and Vrindavan and one of the images we have been given is that of the dance coming to the end; at the final stage all the *Gopis* stand in a circle and between every two *Gopi* girls there is one Krishna. This picturesque view of the *Rasaleela* shows that between two activities – the *Gopi* girls – is the restful Krishna, the *Param-Atman*.

This represents the rest that we ought to have after each activity so that we can initiate the next activity, with a better understanding and a better availability of the forces within us.

As far as the thought process is concerned, the *Sattvic* person just listens and understands the content and form of what is said. The *Rajasic* person does listen sometimes and gets a partial view, while the *Tamasic* person either falls asleep or into a trance and misses everything or forgets very soon whatever he has heard. He holds nothing or misunderstands.

Laws: Cosmic & Individual *(January 1970)*
HH: When one feels the *Ahankar* one always feels a limitation, a circle created by the feeling of *Ahankar*. Whatever happens, whether *Sattvic, Rajasic*, or *Tamasic*, there will have to be some limitation, but these limitations differ by their nature. If *Ahankar* is *Rajasic* or *Tamasic*, it will be related to whatever one thinks of one's body or one's status, one's knowledge or material possessions. So one can come to limit one's *Ahankar* to one's own body or one's own knowledge or good character, or brilliance, or intellect or whatever one seems to have.

These are small circles created by the *Ahankar* and therefore are extremely limited. The other *Ahankar* which is *Sattvic* is related to the *Samashti*. *Samashti* is the Universal Being, the *Param-Atman*. (*Vyashti* is the individual being.) If one accepts the limitations as imposed upon the *Param-Atman*, then one is not possessed by *Rajas* or *Tamas*, is not attached to the action or the outcome that one has grown to associate with performing certain actions. So when the feeling of 'me and mine' arises related to anything in the Universe, this *Ahankar* will be governed by *Rajas* and *Tamas*. On the contrary if the feeling is derived from 'Thee and Thine', then all activities or all vantage grounds to which *Ahankar* rises in any individual, will be of service to him and humanity.

So if one forms the mental attitude that everything available to the individual really belongs to the *Param-Atman*, the individual being only an instrument in performing all his activities, then it will be a *Sattvic Ahankar*. If one thinks that all the situations belong to the Father of All,[†] then the germ of *Rajasic* and *Tamasic Ahankar* will not penetrate the individual, and he will consider himself to be only smaller compared with what has gone before. In the same way, one should always think about all the glory which becomes available to individuals that it will all belong to the *Param-Atman* and we in our activities will just be instrumental in putting this glory into the world. This is the right attitude and by this feeling, the self-pride (false *Ahankar*) will not pervade the individual. Thus one can keep on working on the Ladder of Self-Realisation.

[†]*Mahabharata*, Book 12, Chapter 315, v. 2. Yajnavalkya speaks to Janaka: 'The unmanifest Absolute, by means of the six unions of the gunas (sixfold *yoga* of gunas) transforms himself into hundreds and thousands and millions and millions of forms.'

Faith: Surrendering Buddhi

Question from FCR   (September 1975)
His Holiness says that *Param-Atman* gives to each person what is good for him – what they deserve – and what is good for them. Yet we see all kinds of tragedies around which are difficult to understand, and this drives many people away.

HH: One has to understand the two facets here, one is *Samashti* and the other is *Vyashti*; and the presiding Deity (or the responsible Being) of *Samashti* is the *Param-Atman* himself, and the responsible person of *Vyashti* is the *Jiva*, oneself. There are two sets of laws responsible for the government of these two levels. The set of laws which govern the individual (*Vyashti*) are the outcome of the activities which have been performed by that individual in the cycles of birth and death. The reward for the deeds which he has performed in his previous life will be presented to him in this life. For instance, one might be going along the street and be involved in an accident and fall dead or seriously injured there. Obviously there is nothing to indicate the responsibility of the individual for being knocked down in the street. The only causal explanation that could be given for such accidents is that he may have done something in his previous life for which he is paying the price today, according to his *Prarabdha* (which is unknown to him).

> There was a judge living in Varanasi. Being a well-read person and having been appointed a judge, he did not have much respect for the religious life, nor for the *Param-Atman*, and though living in Varanasi which is the main seat of the Vishwanath, the God Shiva, he never believed in Him so he never went to pay his respects. But his mother was a very religious and dedicated soul – she always tried to impress

on him that he should come with her at least once to the Vishwanath temple. The judge always said he was a busy man with too many things to do. Religious observances were for ignorant people, so they could go and pray to the God, but he would have nothing to do with Him. One Sunday, as he had no business to attend to, his mother again insisted that he should come with her. She pressed him, and finally as an obedient son, he agreed to go with her.

As they were going to the temple in their vehicle, and just before they arrived, there was a crash, and the judge suffered in the accident. He was not badly injured, but despite his slight injuries he became very agitated and blamed his mother for having involved him in this horrible accident which he was not at all ready to accept. He called for a doctor and got his wounds bandaged but then, during the night, he had a dream. In this dream the Lord Shiva appeared Himself and told him, 'You silly man, you were destined to have a big accident, and some of your limbs would have been badly broken. A serious accident was due to befall you because of the misdeeds of your previous life, but because your mother insisted on bringing you to My doors, your sentence was reduced and you were given only a small penalty. Had you not come here this Sunday, you would have been in hospital for months and months.'

When he got up next morning, he went to his mother and apologised, put his head on her feet, and ever after he was a believer, a believer in the existence of God.

This set of laws are there to govern the individual and they will keep on governing. Whatever happens is the reward of one's own deeds. One should understand these laws. Having understood the laws, the misery following any seeming misfortune would be reduced.

Then there are the laws which govern large numbers within the *Samashti* (the Universe). For instance, fifty people may be sitting in a boat and the boat might sink in the river, and one cannot say that all fifty deserve the same fate. There may be one who deserves it or none, but this is at the level of the *Samashti* – there have to be certain accidents. Because of the *Samashti* activity and the *Prarabdha* all these things happen – trains collide and hundreds of people die; a war comes and thousands of people die; at the frontier, the forces from two different nations face each other and shoot and kill each other. This does not come about because of the deeds of the individual – although for everything that happens on either level, payment has to be made by individuals everywhere. The presiding Deity of the *Samashti* is the *Param-Atman* himself but he responds with neither sorrow nor pleasure; so far as he is concerned it is only a play – a drama which is being enacted and he is not involved in the justice of what is being performed, but he must act because the laws are there and his laws must be carried on. Since it comes back to the individual both on the *Vyashti* level and the *Samashti* level, then the need for understanding is doubly necessary.

If one understands these two sets of laws, then one refrains from attaching oneself to whatever results come in life, either by oneself or as part of the universal laws of nature.

Just as in a drama having performed all the different activities, behind the curtain the individual remains the same, having no attachment of any sort, and he does not react to the pleasures or miseries of the drama on the stage. This is all one has to understand. If one understands these two sets of laws and detaches oneself from the resulting miseries and sorrows, then one would simply live according to the laws, both of which are regulated by the *Param-Atman*.

There will never be a time when everything will be going smoothly. In the nature of things there will always be some agitation, for the creation itself is the product of agitation. There will be imbalance all the time. But there is a way to escape from this agitated state of the universe and that has been suggested to you all as in the Meditation, *samadhi* and deep sleep. Having gone deep into Meditation then you come to a state of equilibrium where the laws do not contaminate you – they do not touch you. That is the only moment of equilibrium available, apart from deep sleep, for there will always be disturbances in the Universe and we ought to learn to face them with detachment so that their effect of misery, ecstasy or pleasure does not bind us.

Question from FCR (October 1977)
One seems to jump sometimes from disbelief and despair to a sort of blind belief. So it is hard to see the laws – even the law of cause and effect on this level.

HH: The situation where one jumps from despair and disbelief to blind belief comes from a particular type who relies half on his own judgment. He goes according to what he thinks to be right or wrong, but when he has tried every way he knows and has not succeeded in the work he has undertaken, then he finds no solution and surrenders himself to the *Param-Atman*, to the will of the *Param-Atman*. Whether he really surrenders or not is very difficult to say, but if one could learn to surrender fully to the *Param-Atman*, even after surrender one will have to use one's *Buddhi*. Surrender does not mean that everything will be done for you – you still have to do the work, and it can only be done through the *Buddhi*. The effect of *Buddhi* is that, if it is motivated by the individual's ego, it can perform only limited action. But, if the *Buddhi* is surrendered to the *Param-Atman*, so that *Buddhi* gets its power through the *Param-Atman* then whatever situation arises, the individual who has truly surrendered himself will find that the answers to those questions, those problems, and those incidents will be available, although he may never have given them a thought. This is the way it works.

Question from FCR
HH's diagnosis yesterday remedied the situation where in the half-dream state one jumps from disbelief to blind belief. Certainly it comes from not surrendering fully. And now one very much wants that *Buddhi* should be governed by the *Param-Atman*. But how? One seems to want somebody watching and saying: 'Stop, Doctor! You are at this moment relying on your own judgment and not waiting for the guidance.'

HH: Even this observation comes from *Buddhi*, and when *Buddhi* is united with the *Atman* – whatever action is taken, then if something goes wrong after taking the action one should pray internally to be forgiven, and if the work happens to be right then one should thank the *Param-Atman* for the guidance.

It is essential that the unity between the *Atman* and the *Buddhi*, the internal organs, must take place, and a decision must appear automatically, whether the action which is taken is right or wrong.

This confidence and certainty which comes as a result of the inter-action of *Buddhi* and the promptings from *Atman* must be honoured. Even if, ultimately, it turns out to be wrong this is very important.

> For example, there was a disciple who was given a particular Mantra to worship a Goddess. The proper Mantra was *Kreem*, and the disciple was sounding a Mantra which was connected with Lord Krishna – *Kleem* – very little difference. He went on with this mantra and after some time the Goddess herself appeared and said 'Look here, you are doing your Mantra wrongly – you should change it.' The disciple said how could he believe his Mantra was wrong when it had materialised his Goddess in front of him – if the Mantra was wrong surely the Goddess could never have appeared before him, and he did not change the Mantra but kept on with the way he was saying it, and it is said that the Goddess was pleased.

If this confidence of the *Atman* in unity with the *Buddhi* says that something is right, then it ought to be right whatever happens; if one decides to do something and if one is doing a right thing, yet one feels inside that it is wrong to be done then nothing can make it right – things will go wrong whatever happens, even with the right means. Ultimately it is very difficult to say what is right or wrong! Everything has to be referred to the *Atman*, and if *Atman* says it is right, it is right, and if *Atman* says it is wrong, it will be wrong.

FCR: So, one goes by results – one does what one believes to be right in that state of unity, and goes by results?

HH: With that confidence, the result will always be good.

Question from MA (February 1985)
His Holiness once told us that at any moment, if you listen, *Buddhi* tells you 'yes' or 'no', in relation to the *Param-Atman* and that if you obey this, the voice will get stronger – is this something one can do at any moment?

HH: What comes out of one's *Buddhi* in relation to the problem in hand, or some danger in front of one – *Buddhi* is most careful to try to save the individual, because in saving the individual, *Buddhi* itself is also saved. So one should not think that everything *Buddhi* says is true to the *Param-Atman*. *It depends entirely upon the level of the Buddhi what type of answer you will get.* *Buddhi* certainly gives the answer but the question is, what sort of *Buddhi*?

As far as connecting oneself to the Teacher and trying to get inspiration through the *Buddhi* of the Teacher – in rare conditions this is possible – it is possible to connect directly with the mind of the Teacher if all the necessary conditions are there, but these conditions are rare.

> There was a saint – Vishwanath – and one of his disciples, by meditating constantly on him for a very long time, did reach a state where he was in direct contact with whatever was going on in the mind of the Saint. One day, while Vishwanath was sitting on the bank of the Ganges, he saw that one of his disciples was in great trouble because his boat was caught up in a whirlpool. The Saint did not want him to lose his life. What really happened no one could know, but His whole body was shaking. After some time the boat got out of trouble, with no loss of life. Now the disciple who was standing there said: 'My Teacher, the boat is now safe, why are you still shaking'?

So Vishwanath was startled and said, 'How did you know?' Then the disciple said that he had been meditating on him for a long time, and that eventually he could see everything in his *Antahkarana* – his *Manas*.

Now such a thing is possible, but it is extremely rare – it all depends upon the *Buddhi*. If *Buddhi* is pure, you may be in a pure state for a moment, and then you will get a pure answer – it does not mean that you will always be in a pure state – it may fluctuate, and there may be situations where the circumstances influence the decision and you do not get the right answer. One should not take it for granted that you will always get the right answer.

Question (October 1977)
What is it that surrenders the *Buddhi*?

HH: It is the *Atman* itself, and the *Atman* needs no indication or information about to whom to surrender, because he surrenders to himself. The *Atman* surrenders *Buddhi* to the *Param-Atman*!

Consistency
Question (October 1977)
When the *Chitta* is pure and is open to the *Param-Atman*, can it then be said that the Causal Body operates and controls the Subtle and Physical bodies?

HH: When the *Chitta* is open to the *Param-Atman* it also happens that the *Buddhi* works according to the promptings of the *Atman*, and if this is the situation then everything in the physical body, in the subtle body and the causal body works in response to one order, which means that whatever is done, whatever is said, whatever is thought conforms to one single idea, one order, and in this case, everything is right – everything is controlled at Causal level. If it is only *Manas* and *Ahankar* giving the order to the individual, then it is probable that all the bodies will not fall into line, there will be disparity between what is thought, what is resolved, and what is said and what is done. When one sees that somebody is thinking one thing, saying something else and doing something else again, then this is the act of a man whose *Chitta* is not open to the *Param-Atman*, whose *Buddhi* is not working in conformity with reason, whose *Manas* is not following the dictates of *Buddhi*, and consequently nor does the body. Here is a Sanskrit saying:

> When the thoughts and utterings, whatever one says and does, follow the same thing, then these are the marks of a good man. If they do not correspond to each other, they are the marks of a bad man.

There is a good way to check if the *Chitta* is pure or not. When the *Chitta* is pure and the promptings come from the *Atman*, then the effect of the Causal body on the Subtle body, and the effect of the Subtle body on the physical body is felt, and *seen* to be felt. But if it is the work of *Ahankar* and *Manas*, then there will be no effect from the subtle body on the physical body, rather the other way round – the physical body will affect the subtle body and so on. This is the way one can see if one is following the *Atman* or the *Ahankar*, by whether the internal organs are pure or impure.

Desires

Question (August 1979)

There are different sorts of desires – long desires, short desires, worldly desires and spiritual desires – are these the openings out of the canal which have to be closed through meditation and made into one desire for consciousness?

HH: The realm of desires and their fulfilment is the common realm. Some people have more desires than others and certainly through all the disciplines we can learn to minimise our desires. The more they are minimised the more force of consciousness will be available to use through our desires.

There is a way whereby there is no cessation of activity and yet there is no desire – there is no concept of achievement – there is no entanglement, no attachment to any activity, yet there is a ready response to do whatever nature calls for, whatever the moment demands of you.

This surrender to the activity generated by the nature itself is a state where there is no hankering by the individual – whatever is wanted he picks it up and puts it down instantly when the time to stop has come. He thinks no more about it and he may pick it up later on if he is called upon to do exactly the same thing again. Ordinarily it might seem very odd because in common life most of us like to finish the job because completion of the work is related to achievement – the fulfilment of the desire.

There is an example to see the two in action, for instance when you go to the office to work you reach there by 9.00am and start work, and the moment it is 5 o'clock you stop everything, pack up the papers and go home. But on Saturdays and Sundays, when we are at home and not attending to office work, we do our own work, follow our own pursuits and never look at our watches because we want to complete the activity. Without attending to time we keep on doing the work and if we can't finish the work, if we can't, then the next day we rise again with the same desire to be implemented and it activates us again.

There are desires which are few, there are desires which are many and then there are routine desires like getting up early in the morning and performing certain acts very necessary for the health of the individual, or for daily work.

Common man does not know that there is a way where there is no desire and yet the day is full of activity. Judges seem to have this capacity – when they go into Court they have no thought about the cases – the case is put before them, they listen to it with great attention, give their ruling or sentence – whatever is necessary and, having done so, they leave the Court without having any further worries about the case, and they can keep on doing this day after day without any involvement.

It is the *involvement* which we have to learn to give up – if our attachments are given up then we can reach a state where we should be able to be active and do all our work without any loss of consciousness, without any loss of energy – no sense of achievement and no fulfilment of desire.

Sacrifice and Surrender *(January 1991)*
Would His Holiness say more about sacrifice. Is it the final surrender, full of happiness and joy, of one's attitude to worldly attractions and is it needed to know always that *Atman* is my real Self. Is it a once and final sacrifice or does one have to do it regularly?

HH: Sacrifice is an important factor of spiritual discipline for realisation of the *Atman* or liberation. By liberation it is meant that the *Atman* is liberated from possessions and attachments. When *Atman* alone remains then it shines in its full glory and needs nothing else.

Sacrifices are of two types: internal and external. The worldly possessions which one acquires and hoards for continuous and constant pleasure are the subject of external sacrifice. All that is the source of pleasure comes with attachment and so is an object of bondage, a hindrance to Self-realisation.

Sacrifice is a gradual process and each time it makes one lighter in two ways; it enlightens, and it lightens the burden. Those who desire to realize the *Atman* have to sacrifice all their burdens on the way. Sacrifice is to reach out to help others in need. Possessions are for relishing at moments of one's choice at the expense of others.

Internal sacrifice is equally important. Within each *Antahkarana* there lie valued possessions of love, hate, attachments, desires, anger, greed, pride, prejudice and *ahankaras* of various types. These too need to be sacrificed to unload the mind and purify one's *Antahkarana*. These are subtle possessions and they are hard to part with. The ultimate realization is to have nothing else but the *Atman*, so everything else must go. One cannot sacrifice the *Atman* for it is limitless and One, without any 'second' to receive it. Internal and external sacrifices make one light and with lightness one feels free. A boat carrying a heavy burden sinks deep in the water and moves very slowly. A lighter boat floats freely and moves faster to reach its destination. What belongs to the individual is all subject to sacrifice or surrender.

In worldly life, if one comes under certain influences such as the scriptures, the teacher, a wise man or some moment of heightened experience one may easily resolve to sacrifice everything; but to put that resolution into practice is difficult without proper understanding of the philosophical reasoning. Possessions are for pleasure and pleasure comes from things outside oneself. Bliss comes from within when there are no possessions. This is the form of *Sat Chit Ananda*. Truth, Consciousness and Bliss arise by themselves. Sacrifice leads to that state where bliss can arise in the full consciousness of *Atman*, which is the true creator of all the glorious things in creation. By sacrifice one loses nothing but gains the *Param-Atman*. *Prakriti* (Nature) carries on worldly affairs, the drama unfolds scene by scene and the witness, the *Atman*, remains in bliss. This is also the state of *Sthitaprajna*. He ascends and holds to the centre where there is nothing but that which is the cause of all things. Both external and internal possessions have to be sacrificed gradually. The final sacrifice is the *Ahankara* of sacrifice itself and then what remains is Truth, Consciousness and Bliss, the Self – Advaita.

Sthitaprajna *(November 1973)*
HH: The ultimate end of meditation is to reach to this total immobility, or profound stillness, and this is very deep. No meter could measure it; it is without end. It is not necessary that one should remain in this state for a long period. Longer meditation does not mean the achievement of this profound stillness. Most of the time spent during the meditation is in preparation to lead one to this state. There may be meditators who sit for hours and hours to no avail, for they keep on churning their mechanical thoughts in habitual rotation. They end up tired, both physically and mentally. Those who manage to dive deep, they come out with potentiality emanating from the Will of the Absolute.

During the *Mahabharata* episode Arjuna asked Shri Krishna about the man with such stillness. In the *Gita*, such a man is called *Sthitaprajna* (one who is steady and still in his Knowledge and Being). Krishna says that such a man does not become agitated by discomfort, pain or misery. He does not rise in revolt against misfortune. Even if calamity befalls, he neither gives up nor feels regret – he attends only to overcoming its effects with a smile. When honoured with success, pleasure, or comforts he never bursts into jubilation; he simply accepts with gratitude, and then forgets. In short, one could say that a man with this profound stillness always remains the same and expresses efficiency, wisdom, love and mercy.

Extract from a letter from Shri Narayan Swaroop
(January 1978)
His Holiness says that a mother never bothers how dirty her child is. She just washes the child and takes him up into her arms. Similarly the Lord never bothers about what condition we are in, whether we are clean in our hearts or not, He is ready to clean us if only we would let Him do so. The difficulty is that we do not even let Him do so, our ego stands in the way.

His Holiness says that all we have to do is just repeat His Name, which means remembering His qualities. The rest He will do Himself. The Name is full of power, its repetition does the trick, It generates faith and creates a longing desire, This in turn cleans our hearts and leads us to the ultimate goal. Complete surrender means a positive and deep faith that nothing is possible except by His Grace. This is not shifting one's burden to someone else, but to me this is the absolute truth. This line of thought will not lead anyone to inactivity because He knows our needs and will not let us sit idle. He will create circumstances which will make us act in a much better way than we could achieve by our own will.

When asked how one can increase one's love for the Lord, His Holiness has often advised to go on just repeating the Mantra, the Name that the Guru has given. This in itself will generate faith which will enable one to leave the rest of one's advancement to Him. His Holiness insists that we should continue recitation of the Name. He says that a stage will come when we can do without the recitation. It will become part of one Being, one's very existence. We have nothing else to do.

His Holiness often stresses that we do not need to worry about purification of the heart. We cannot gain it by our own efforts, but if we continue with the recitation it will be a natural corollary. Name reminds one of the qualities of the Name. The Lord above all, all mercy, He is present with us always. Wherever we may be, He knows what is best for us, and what is more He is so merciful that He is always ready to give it to us and make us worthy to deserve, to get what is best for us.

INDEX

As 'Param-Atman' occurs so frequently throughout this book
it has not been included in the index.

150

The Study Society

The Study Society offers a variety of courses, activities and study groups for anyone deeply attracted to the practical possibilities of self-development and Self-realisation. Introductory courses are available for those who wish to understand more of the Shankaracharya's teaching and to work with others on its daily practice. These are supported by a unique and extensive record of questions and answers given over 30 years by the Shankaracharya to members of the Society. The Society provides several other complementary approaches to the experience of the fundamental Unity of creation with the individual, including knowledge and methods from the Sufi tradition and the Fourth Way system of P D Ouspensky and Francis Roles.

Meditation is for many an essential method in following this path. For more than 50 years the Society has provided training in a simple technique of mantra meditation designed to allow a daily connection with the real Self – the source of inner peace, understanding and happiness that is the foundation for every individual's search for truth and Unity.

Activities and study groups take place at our headquarters in West London and at various locations around the UK. We also have affiliated organisations around the world. Please see our website for details.

The Study Society
Colet House
151 Talgarth Road, London W14 9DA
020 8741 6568
www.studysociety.org
office@studysociety.org